CNA Book For The State Exam

1000 Review Questions for

The Nursing Assistant Test Preparation

Key Points Exam Prep Team

CNA Book for the state exam
1000 Review Questions for the Nursing Assistant Test Preparation

www.healthcarebooks.ORG

ISBN-13: 978-1983557248

ISBN-10: 1983557242

Printed in the United States of America.

Section 1

Introduction to care agencies

1. Which of the following is a type of healthcare agency?
   a. Clinics
   b. Memory care facilities
   c. Drug and alcohol treatment center
   d. All of the above
2. Which of the following is part of health promotion?
   a. Immunization
   b. Physical examination
   c. Counseling about health living
   d. Emergency care
3. The goal of health promotion is to ....
   a. Reduce risk of mental illness
   b. Return the person to their highest possible level of physical functioning
   c. Prevent disease
   d. Treat disease
4. Detection and treatment of disease involves ....
   a. Immunization
   b. Surgery
   c. Teaching about diet
   d. All of the above
5. Rehabilitation process starts when ....
   a. The person first seeks health care
   b. The person takes the first drug
   c. The person takes the first injection
   d. All of the above
6. Which of the following is done in restorative care?
   a. The person learns skills needed to live, work and enjoy life
   b. The is admitted to the emergency department
   c. The person is examined
   d. The person is observed for signs and symptoms
7. ....is a sudden illness from which the person is expected to recover
   a. Chronic illness
   b. Terminal illness
   c. Acute illness
   d. Minor illness
8. ......is an illness or injury from which the person will not likely recover
   a. Chronic illness
   b. Terminal illness

c. Acute illness

d. Major illness

9. Which of the following service is provided in the hospital?

   a. Laboratory test

   b. X-ray procedures

   c. Nursing care

   d. All of the above

10. Persons in long term care are called ......

    a. Patients

    b. Residents

    c. In-patients

    d. Inmates

11. Which of the following is true about long-term care center?

    a. All persons in the long-term centers are old

    b. Persons admitted in long-term care centers still need hospital care

    c. Persons in long-term care centers cannot care for themselves

    d. All of the above

12. An assisted living residence provides which of the following?

    a. Personal care

    b. Health care

    c. Support services

    d. All of the above

13. ....is a health care agency or program for persons who are dying

    a. Home care agencies

    b. Hospices

    c. Assisted living residence

    d. Mental health care centers

14. Which of the following is true about health care systems?

    a. It is all usually covered by most insurance

    b. It does not include a hospice center

    c. Agencies join together as one provider of care

    d. All of the above

15. An agency has a governing body called ....

    a. Board of trustees

    b. Managers

    c. Directors of nursing

    d. Medical director

16. Which of the following manages the agency?

    a. Administrator

    b. Business director

    c. Director of nursing

    d. Board of directors

17. Which of the following is part of the health team?
    a. Cleric
    b. Homemaker
    c. Dentist
    d. All of the above

18. ....prevents the disease of the gums
    a. Licensed practical nurse
    b. Home health aide
    c. Dentist
    d. Dietitian

19. ....prevents, diagnoses and treat foot disorders
    Physician
    Podiatrist
    Pharmacist
    Nursing assistants

20. ....is responsible for the entire nursing staffs
    a. Administrator
    b. Director of nursing
    c. Nurse practitioner
    d. Licensed vocational nurse

21. Which of the following is a responsibility of the charge nurse?
    a. Coordinates nursing care for a certain shift
    b. They are responsible for all the nursing staffs
    c. Provides nursing care in a nursing specialty
    d. Implements recreational needs

22. A registered nurse has completed a ....nursing program and has passed the licensing test
    a. 3 years university program
    b. 1 year hospital based diploma program
    c. 2 years community college program
    d. 4 years community college program

23. Which of the following is a part of the nursing team?
    a. Physician
    b. Nursing assistant
    c. Social worker
    d. Dentist

24. A licensed practical nurse has completed .... and has passed a licensing test
    a. 3 year diploma
    b. 4 years university degree
    c. 1 year nursing program
    d. 2 months vocational training

25. Which of the following is a function of a nursing assistant?
   a. Give treatment
   b. Give baths
   c. Give drugs
   d. All of the above
26. Which of the following is a case manager?
   a. Registered nurse
   b. Nursing assistant
   c. Licensed vocational nurse
   d. Physician
27. ....is bought by individuals and families
   a. Group insurance
   b. Medicaid
   c. Medicare
   d. Private insurance
28. Medicare is for persons ....or older
   a. 50
   b. 55
   c. 60
   d. 65
29. Which of the following is true about Medicare?
   a. There is no monthly insurance premium
   b. It is often an employee benefit
   c. The person pays for monthly premium
   d. It is only for old people
30. Part A of medicare pays for which of the following care?
   a. Home care cost
   b. Occupational therapist
   c. Out patient hospital care
   d. Physical therapist
31. Medicare severity adjusted diagnosis related groups are for ....
   a. Rehabilitation centers
   b. Home health care
   c. Hospital cost
   d. All of the above
32. Which of the following is true about prospective payment systems?
   a. If the cost of treatment is greater than the amount paid, the agency is paid the balance
   b. If the cost of treatment is less than the amount paid the agency takes the extra money
   c. The amount paid for the services is determined after treatment

d. If the cost of treatment is less than the amount paid the agency refunds the extra money

33. Case mix groups are used for ....
    a. Home health resource groups
    b. Rehabilitation centers
    c. SNF payments
    d. Hospital costs

34. Which of the following is true about managed care?
    a. It limits the choice of where to go for health care
    b. Health care services must be preapproved before services are used
    c. The insurer decides what to pay for
    d. All of the above

35. Healthcare standards are set by ......
    a. Federal governments
    b. State governments
    c. Accrediting agencies
    d. All of the above

36. ....is required to receive Medicare and Medicaid funds
    a. Licensure
    b. Certification
    c. Accreditation
    d. All of the above

37. ....is voluntary, it signals quality and excellence
       License
       Approval
      Accreditation
      Certification

38. Which of the following will the survey team do?
    a. Review medical records
    b. Observe how care is given
    c. Review budgets and finances
    d. All of the above

39. The agency is usually given ....days to correct a deficiency
    a. 1 week
    b. 2 weeks
    c. 60 days
    d. 1 year

40. Which of the following should be done when filling a survey?
    a. Be honest
    b. Do not rush
    c. Finish and return in a timely manner
    d. All of the above

Section 2

The person's rights

1. Which of the following explains the person's rights and expectations during hospital stays?
    a. The patient care partnership: Understanding expectations, rights, and responsibilities
    b. Health insurance portability and accountability Act
    c. Protected health information
    d. All of the above

2. The omnibus budget reconciliation act is a ....
    a. Federal law
    b. State law
    c. American hospital association act
    d. Hospital policy

3. Which of the following is expected during a person's stay at the hospital?
    a. A clean environment
    b. High quality hospital care
    c. A safe environment
    d. All of the above

4. The patient should know which of the following?
    a. The benefits and risk of each treatment
    b. Whether the treatment is experimental
    c. What to expect from the treatment
    d. All of the above

5. Residents who are incompetent has a .... who act on their behalf
    a. Lawyer
    b. Representative
    c. Advocate
    d. Jury

6. Request for information should be passed to the ....
    a. Nurse
    b. Doctor
    c. Administrator
    d. Board of trustees

7. ....are written instructions about healthcare when a person is not able to make such decisions a. Wills
    b. Testament
    c. Advance directives
    d. Memorial documentation

8. Privacy can be protected by ....

a. Removing the resident from public view

b. Providing clothes to prevent unnecessary exposure

c. Closing curtains

d. All of the above

9. Which of the following is a right of the resident?

To share a room with his or her spouse

To closet space

To refuse treatment

All of the above

10. Which of the following should be done when a resident is making a call?

a. Leave the room

b. Sit down

c. Give oral hygiene

d. Clean the room

11. The ....decides when to eat

a. Registered nurse

b. Nursing assistant

c. Patient

d. Doctor

12. Which of the following is a form of involuntary seclusion?

a. Keeping the person in a certain area

b. Depriving the person of goods needed to attain well being

c. Willful inflict of injury

d. Punishment that results in physical harm

13. The agency cannot employ which of the following people?

a. A person older than 50

b. A person younger than 21

c. A person found guilty of abusing others

d. All of the above

14. A center must make changes when a resident ....

a. Is getting older

b. Is sick

c. Is worried about falling

d. Losses a loved one

15. Long term care ombudsmen are employed by ....

a. Federal agency

b. State agency

c. Hospital

d. American hospital association

Section 3

The nursing assistant

1. Which of the following occurred prior to 1980?
    a. Nursing assistants were required to train by law
    b. Primary nursing was not common
    c. Many hospitals hire only RNs
    d. All of the above

2. Which of the following was done in other to reduce hospital cost?
    a. Hospital closures
    b. Hospital mergers
    c. Health care systems
    d. All of the above

3. A nurse practice act does which of the following?
    a. Defines RN and LPN/LVN
    b. Describes education and licensing requirements for RNs
    c. Protects the public from persons practicing without a license
    d. All of the above

4. ....is used to determine what the nursing assistant can do
    a. State nurse practice act
    b. Federal law
    c. Job description
    d. Hospital policy

5. OBRA requires at least .... Hours of instruction as requirement for nursing assistants
    a. 25
    b. 65
    c. 75
    d. 100

6. Which of the following is contained in the nursing assistant registry?
    a. Date of birth
    b. Height
    c. Parent's occupation
    d. Insurance details

7. Re-training is required for nursing assistant who have not worked for ....
    a. 12 months
    b. 24 months
    c. 6 months
    d. 36 months

8. Which of the following is a reason to have your licensed revoked?
    a. Substance abuse

b. Giving unsafe care

c. Violating a person's privacy

d. All of the above

9. Which of the following function does a nursing assistant perform?

   a. Gives drug

   b. Take oral orders from doctors

   c. Assist a nurse with sterile technique

   d. Supervise other nursing assistants

10. ....is responsible for all nursing care

   a. Registered nurse

   b. Licensed nurse

   c. Nursing assistant

   d. Administrator

11. Which of the following should be understood before accepting a job?

   a. Sterilizing techniques

   b. Your job description

   c. Surgical procedures

   d. All of the above

12. ....cannot delegate nursing tasks

   a. RN

   b. LVN

   c. LPN

   d. Nursing assistant

13. The first step in the delegation process is to ....

   a. Assess

   b. Communicate

   c. Supervise

   d. Evaluate

14. Which of the following is one of the five rights to delegation?

   a. The right time

   b. The right task

   c. The right patient

   d. The right place

15. A task can be refused when ....

   a. You are tired

   b. You are busy

   c. You were not prepared to perform the task

   d. You are unhappy

Section 4

Ethics and laws

1. ....is the knowledge of what is right conduct and wrong conduct
   a. Morals
   b. Ethics
   c. Law
   d. All of the above

2. Judgment and views are based on the person's........
   a. Culture
   b. Religion
   c. Education
   d. All of the above

3. ....separates helpful behaviors from behaviors that are not helpful
   a. Professional boundaries
   b. Accreditation
   c. Barriers
   d. Professional ethics

4. ....is a brief act or behavior outside of the helpful zone
   a. Professional sexual misconduct
   b. Assault
   c. Boundary violation
   d. Boundary crossing

5. Which of the following is an act of boundary crossing?
   a. Giving a crying patient a hug
   b. Abusing the person sexually
   c. Keeping secrets
   d. Telling a person about your personal relationships

6. Which of the following must be done to maintain professional boundaries?
   a. Do not date residents
   b. Do not use offensive language
   c. Do not help them with finances
   d. All of the above

7. Which of the following is a boundary sign?
   a. The person gives you money
   b. You flirt with the person
   c. You give the person gifts
   d. All of the above

8. Which of the following is an unintentional tort?
   a. Malpractice
   b. Defamation
   c. Slander
   d. Libel

9. ....is an unintentional wrong
    a. Malpractice
    b. Negligence
    c. Libel
    d. Slander

10. ....is negligence by a professional person
    a. Fraud
    b. Assault
    c. Malpractice
    d. Mistake

11. Which of the following could lead to charges of negligence
    a. Failure to test water temperature before hot soak
    b. Delay in answering signal light
    c. Not following manufacturers instruction
    d. All of the above

12. .... is making false statement in print, writing or through pictures
    a. Accusation
    b. Libel
    c. Slander
    d. Abuse

13. ....is intentionally attempting or threatening to touch a person's body without the person's consent a. Battery
    b. Invasion of privacy
    c. Assault
    d. Defamation

14. A person under the age of .... cannot give consent
    a. 18
    b. 21
    c. 16
    d. 10

15. Which of the following is a role of a nursing assistant as regards the will of a patient?
    a. You can help draft the will
    b. You may witness the signing
    c. You can proof read the will
    d. All of the above

16. .... Is a legal document of how the person wants property distributed after
death
    a. Written consent
    b. Notice
    c. Will

d. Advance directive
17. Which of the following is a form of abuse?
   a. Willful infliction of injury
   b. Unreasonable confinement
   c. Punishment that results in physical harm
   d. All of the above
18. Which of the following can be an abuser?
   a. Caregiver
   b. Spouse
   c. Adult child
   d. All of the above
19. Which of the following is a form of physical abuse?
   a. Sneering at the person
   b. Hair pulling
   c. Threats
   d. All of the above
20. Which of the following is a type of emotional abuse?
   a. Humiliation
   b. Involuntary seclusion
   c. Neglect
   d. Corporal punishment

Section 5

Work ethics

1. Work ethics involves ………
   a. How you look
   b. What you say
   c. How you behave
   d. All of the above
2. Which of the following should be avoided?
   a. Salty foods
   b. Sleep
   c. Exercise
   d. All of the above
3. Which of the following should be done to maintain personal hygiene?
   a. Take 7 hours of sleep
   b. Use deodorant
   c. Regular exercise

d. Regular medical checkup

4. Jobs can be found through ....
   a. Internet
   b. Newspaper ads
   c. The clinical experience site
   d. All of the above

5. The nursing assistant when on duty should wear which of the following?
   a. Jewelry in pierced nose
   b. Perfume
   c. Undergarments
   d. Nail polish

6. Which of the following qualities should a nursing assistant portray?
   a. Honesty
   b. Should be courteous
   c. Should be respectful
   d. All of the above

7. Being eager and excited about your work is being ....
   a. Courteous
   b. Enthusiastic
   c. Respectful
   d. Trustworthy

8. Which of the following should be avoided when completing a job application?
   a. Reporting felony arrest
   b. Talking bad about your former employer
   c. Bad writing
   d. Lying on application

9. Which of the following should be done during interview?
   a. Sit with good posture
   b. Avoiding eye contact
   c. Turn on your phone
   d. All of the above

10. Which of the following dressing is appropriate for an interview?
    a. Wearing jeans and shorts
    b. Heavy perfumes
    c. Applying simple makeup
    d. Wearing multiple sets of earrings

11. Which of the following is done by a preceptor?
    a. Introduces you to patients
    b. Helps you review your job description
    c. Helps you review your pay rate and working hours
    d. Supervises your work continually

12. Which of the following should be done to avoid gossiping?
    a. Remove yourself from a group where people are gossiping
    b. Talk about patients only at home
    c. Make hurtful comments to only staff member
    d. All of the above
13. Making a false statement about another person is ………
    a. Abuse
    b. Defamation
    c. Assault
    d. Battery
14. Which of the following should be done when talking?
    a. Using swear words
    b. Yelling
    c. Speaking softly
    d. Using slangs
15. Which of the following can be used to reduce or cope with stress?
    a. Getting enough rest
    b. Eating healthy
    c. Taking a hot bath
d.   All of the above

Section 6

Communicating with the health team

1. Which of the following should be done when communicating with the health team?
    a. Use words with more than one meaning
    b. Use familiar words
    c. Add unrelated information
    d. All of the above
2. ………is a written or electronic account of a person's condition and response to treatment
    a. Medical record
    b. Admission record
    c. Progress note
    d. Graphic sheet
3. ……..is a legal record
    a. X-ray report

b. Medical report

c. Admission report

d. Consultation report

4. If you are not involved in a person's care, viewing the person's chart is ……….

    a. A breach of contract

    b. A defamation

    c. An invasion of privacy

    d. A fraudulent act

5. Which of the following information is included in a person's admission record

    a. Place of worship

    b. Religion

    c. Employer

    d. All of the above

6. Which of the following information is contained in the health history?

    a. Religion

    b. Place of worship

    c. Current drugs

    d. All of the above

7. ……..describes the care given and the person's response and progress

    a. Nursing plan

    b. Progress note

    c. Admission record

    d. Flow sheets

8. ……….summarizes information in the medical record, drugs, treatments, diagnoses, routine care measures, equipment, and special needs a. Kardex

    b. Flow sheets

    c. Progress notes

    d. Graphic sheets

9. Which of the following information is contained in the progress note?

    a. Marital status

    b. Information about treatment and drugs

    c. Allergies

    d. Childhood illness

10. Which of the following should be done when recording?

    a. Use your own abbreviation

    b. Use ditto marks

    c. Record what you observed

    d. Record interpretations

11. Which of the following rules should be followed when recording?

    a. Chart a procedure, or care measure before it is completed

    b. Use terms with more than one meaning

c. Do not omit information

d. All of the above

12. The .... is the word element that contains the basic meaning of the word

   a. Root

   b. Prefix

   c. Suffix

   d. Vowel

13. Voiding is known as ....

   a. Urinating

   b. Spitting

   c. Eating

   d. Sleeping

14. Which of the following should be observed when using the agency's computer and other electronic devices?

   a. Do not tell anyone the username or password

   b. Do not write down or expose username and password

   c. Log off after entry

   d. All of the above

15. Which of the following should be done in case of conflict?

   a. Talk privately with the individual

   b. Explain the problem and what is bothering you

   c. Listen to the person

   d.   All of the above

Section 7

Assisting with the nursing process

1. Which of the following is done during the assessment stage?

   a. The patient is observed

   b. The health problem is treated

   c. Actions to be taken are documented

   d. Documented plans are carried out 2. Through touch you ....

   a. See how the person lies

   b. Listen to how the person breathes

   c. Feel if the skin is hot or cold

   d. All of the above

3. Which of the following is an objective sign?

   a. Pale skin

b. Redness on skin

c. Fear

d. Irregular pulse

4. Which of the following should be reported at once?

   a. Vomiting

   b. Bleeding

   c. Abnormal respirations

   d. All of the above

5. ....is the identification of a disease or condition by a doctor

   a. Medical diagnosis

   b. Nursing observation

   c. Medical assessment

   d. Medical observation

6. Which of the following is an approved nursing diagnosis by the north American nursing diagnosis association international a. Sleep deprivation

   b. Diabetes

   c. Cancer

   d. Fever

7. Which of the following is true about nursing interventions?

   a. It needs a doctor's order

   b. It is chosen before goals are set

   c. It is also known as nursing action

   d. All of the above

8. OBRA requires ...... types of resident care conferences

   a. 2

   b. 3

   c. 4

   d. 5

9. Care is given in the .... stage

   a. Assessment

   b. Nursing diagnosis

   c. Planning

   d. Implementation

10. The assignment sheet does which of the following?

    a. Tells you each person's care

    b. Tells you what nursing tasks to do

    c. Tells you what measure and tasks needs to be done

    d. All of the above

Section 8

Understanding the person

1. The........is the most important person in the agency
   a. Resident
   b. Registered nurse
   c. Nursing assistant
   d. Administrator
2. A whole person has .... part
   a. Spiritual
   b. Physical
   c. Social
   d. All of the above
3. A person should be addressed by his or her ....
   a. Room number
   b. Title and last name
   c. First name
   d. Nickname
4. Which of the following is the lowest level of the human needs?
   a. Self esteem needs
   b. Love and belonging
   c. Physical needs
   d. Safety and security
5. Which of the following is a physical need?
   a. Oxygen
   b. Food
   c. Water
   d. All of the above
6. A woman who has cancer and no longer feels beautiful needs which of the following?
   a. Love and belonging
   b. Self esteem
   c. Self actualization
   d. Water
7. Which of the following is the highest need on the Maslow's hierarchy?
   a. Safety and security needs
   b. Love and belonging
   c. Self actualization
   d. Physical needs

8. Rubbing the skin with a coin to treat cold is common among the ....
   a. Vietnamese
   b. Americans
   c. British
   d. Mexicans

9. ....is a common response to illness and disability
   a. Acceptance
   b. Anger
   c. Helplessness
   d. Hopefulness

10. Which of the following will help bring the patient to the optimal level of function
    a. Encouraging the person to be as independent as possible
    b. Focusing on the disability
    c. Promoting the sick role
    d. All of the above

11. ....is the branch of medicine concerned with the care of women during pregnancy
    a. Pediatrics
    b. Bariatrics
    c. Obstetrics
    d. Geriatrics

12. Psychiatry is the branch of medicine concerned with ....
    a. Mental health problems
    b. Medical problems
    c. Care and development of the brain
    d. Controlling obesity

13. Morbid obesity means that the person weighs ....or more over his or her normal weight a. 40
    b. 50
    c. 100
    d. 150

14. Life threatening problems are referred to which of the following unit?
    a. Special care unit
    b. Pediatric unit
    c. Bariatric
    d. Obstetric

15. Which of the following should be done when communicating with a person?
    a. Avoid medical terms
    b. Be brief
    c. Use words that have the same meaning to both of you
    d. All of the above

16. When communicating with a person ……….
    a. Repeat what you have said
    b. Continue repeating the same exact words till the person understands
    c. Tell the person you are repeating information
    d. Give lengthy explanations
17. When communicating verbally, do not ………..
    a. Speak clearly
    b. Repeat information
    c. Shout
    d. Face the person directly
18. Which of the following is a form of body language?
    a. Shouting
    b. Reading
    c. Gestures
    d. Whispering
19. A constant stare whereby face muscles do not move shows ………
    a. Coldness
    b. Fear
    c. Disgust
    d. Approval
20. In the American culture eye contact signals ……..
    a. Shyness
    b. Openness
    c. Humility
    d. Embarrassment

Section 9

Body structure and function

1. The basic unit of the body structure is the ……..
    a. Cell
    b. DNA
    c. Cytoplasm
    d. Blood
2. Each cell has ……chromosomes
    a. 20
    b. 46
    c. 57

d. 64

3. Group of cells with similar functions combine to form.........
    a. Tissues
    b. Nerves
    c. Systems
    d. Organ

4. ....receives and carries impulses to the brain and back to the body parts
    a. Epithelial tissue
    b. Connective tissue
    c. Nerve tissue
    d. Muscle tissue

5. Systems are formed by ....that work together to perform special functions
    a. Tissues
    b. Nerves
    c. Organs
    d. Cells

6. Which of the following is the largest system?
    a. Integumentary system
    b. Musculo skeletal system
    c. Nervous system
    d. Central nervous system

7. The human body has ....bones
    a. 130
    b. 206
    c. 300
    d. 301

8. Flat bones are at the ....
    a. Legs
    b. Ribs
    c. Spinal column
    d. Fingers

9. ......allows turning from side to side
    a. Pivot joint
    b. Hinge joint
    c. Ball and socket joint
    d. All of the above

10. Muscles attached to the ..... are voluntary muscles
    a. Stomach
    b. Blood vessels
    c. Bones
    d. Heart

11. Which of the following is a function of the muscle?

a. For body movement
b. To maintain good posture
c. Production of body heat
d. All of the above

12. A ……..is anything that excites or causes a body part to function
a. Reflex
b. Stimulus
c. Nerves
d. Impulse

13. All of the following is true about nerves EXCEPT
a. It connects to the spinal cord
b. It is easily damaged
c. It heals quickly
d. It carries messages to the brain

14. Which of the following is the largest part of the brain?
a. Cerebrum
b. Cerebellum
c. Brainstem
d. Pons

15. Which of the following is a function of the cerebellum?
a. It controls speech
b. It regulates body movement
c. It regulates sensation
d. It controls vision

16. The ……….controls heart rate
a. Pons
b. Cerebellum
c. Medulla
d. Spinal cords

17. …….protects the central nervous system
a. Dura matter
b. Arachnoid
c. Pai matter
d. Cerebrospinal fluid

18. The peripheral nervous system has ……pairs of cranial nerves
a. 6
b. 12
c. 24
d. 36

19. Cranial nerves conduct impulses for ……..
a. Smell
b. Vision

c. Hearing

d. All of the above

20. The peripheral nerves controls which of the following body functions?

a. Heartbeat

b. Blood pressure

c. Intestinal contractions

d. All of the above

21. Receptors for taste are in the ....

a. Saliva

b. Tongue

c. Ears

d. Lips

22. The .... is the outer part of the eye

a. Sclera

b. Choroid

c. Retina

d. Cornea

23. Light enters the eye through ....

a. Vitreous humor

b. Aqueous chamber

c. Cornea

d. Retina

24. Which of the following is in the outer part of the ear?

a. Pinna

b. Eardrum

c. Cochlea

d. Saccule

25. Which of the following is part of the circulatory system?

a. Brain

b. Heart

c. Spinal cord

d. Nerves

26. Which of the following is a function of the circulatory system?

a. The blood carries food to the cells

b. The blood removes waste products from the cell

c. The blood transport the gases of respiration

d. All of the above

27. ....carries oxygen to the cells

a. Leukocytes

b. Plasma

c. Hemoglobin

d. Thrombocytes

28. Platelets are formed in the …………

    a. Bone marrow

    b. Plasma

    c. Red blood cells

    d. Blood

29. A platelet lives for about …….

    a. 2 days

    b. 4 days

    c. 1 week

    d. 2 weeks

30. Which of the following is the outer layer of the heart?

    a. Endocardium

    b. Myocardium

    c. Pericardium

    d. None of the above

31. Which of the following occurs in the systole phase of the heart?

    a. The heart is resting

    b. The heart chamber is filled with blood

    c. The heart contracts

    d. All of the above

32. ………. Is the largest artery

    a. Vein

    b. Aorta

    c. Arteriole

    d. Capillaries

33. ……..picks up waste products

    a. Capillaries

    b. Veins

    c. Arteries

    d. Aorta

34. Lymph nodes are shaped like …….

    a. Corn

    b. Rice

    c. Beans

    d. Oranges

35. The right lymphatic nodes collects lymph from the ……..

    a. Right arm

    b. Pelvis

    c. Lower chest

    d. Stomach

36. The ……..is the largest structure in the lymphatic system

    a. Tonsils

b. Adenoids

c. Thymus

d. Spleen

37. Which of the following is a function of the spleen?

   a. It destroys old red blood cells

   b. It filters and removes bacteria

   c. It saves the iron found in hemoglobin when RBCs are destroyed

   d. All of the above

38. ....prevents food from entering the airway during swallowing

   a. Pharynx

   b. Larynx

   c. Epiglottis

   d. Trachea

39. Each lung is covered by ………

   a. Pleura

   b. Sternum

   c. Lymph

   d. Alveoli

40. The …… cut, chop and grind food into small particles

   a. Gum

   b. Tongue

   c. Teeth

   d. Saliva

41. …….absorbs food into the capillaries

   a. Jejunum

   b. Villi

   c. Ileum

   d. Duodenum

42. Which of the following is the function of the urinary system?

   a. It removes waste products from the blood

   b. It maintains water balance within the body

   c. It maintains electrolyte balance

   d. All of the above

43. A pH of …… is neutral

   a. 5

   b. 7

   c. 8

   d. 9

44. The …….produce clear, colorless fluid before ejaculation

   a. Cowper's glands

   b. Vas deferens

   c. Epididymis

d. Scrotum

45. The ……. Is a rounded, fatty pad over a bone called the symphysis pubis
    a. Clitoris
    b. Mons pubis
    c. Labia minora
    d. Labia majora

46. The main part of the uterus is the ……
    a. Cervix
    b. Endometrium
    c. Fundus
    d. Fallopian tubes

47. The pancreas secretes ……….
    a. Insulin
    b. Oxytocin
    c. Thyroxine
    d. Parathormone

48. ………regulates the amount of salt and water that is absorbed and lost by the kidney
    a. Glucocorticoids
    b. Mineralocorticoids
    c. Gonads
    d. None of the above

49. ……….are white blood cells that digest and destroy microorganisms
    a. Lymphocytes
    b. Antigens
    c. Phagocytes
    d. Antibodies

50. ……..causes the production of antibodies that circulates the plasma
    a. T lymphocytes
    b. B lymphocytes
    c. Phagocytes
    d. Antigens

Section 10

Growth and development

1. Growth can be measured in ……….
    a. Height
    b. Weight

   c. Changes in body appearance

   d. All of the above

2. Which of the following is true about growth and development?

   a. Development relates to changes in body functions

   b. Stages of growth do not overlap

   c. Stages of development overlap

   d. All of the above

3. The process of growth and development begins at ....

   a. Fertilization

   b. Birth

   c. The age of 1

   d. At 1 month after birth

4. The process of growth and development ends at ....

   a. Menopause

   b. The age of 90

   c. At the age of 200

   d. Death

5. Which of the following is true about a baby's development and growth?

   a. They hold up their heads before they sit

   b. They control hand movement before shoulder movement

   c. They run before walking

   d. They stand before sitting

6. Which of the following is true about infancy?

   a. Growth and development is slow in the first year of life

   b. They start learning how to eat solid food

   c. They gain control of bowel and bladder function

   d. They use words to communicate

7. Which of the following is true about newborn babies?

   a. The central nervous system is not well developed

   b. Movement lacks purpose and coordination

   c. They can see clearly up to about 8 inches

   d. All of the above

8. .... Occurs when a baby is startled by a loud noise, a sudden movement or the head falling back a. Rooting reflex

   b. Moro reflex

   c. Sucking reflex

   d. Step reflex

9. Newborns sleep for about .... hours a day

   a. 6

   b. 12

   c. 17

   d. 24

10. Which of the following occurs in toddlerhood?
    a. They start to crawl
    b. They begin to get curious
    c. They use gestures to communicate
    d. They babble, coo and gurgle

11. Which of the following is a characteristic of a toddler?
    a. They are very possessive
    b. They scream and kick to express anger and frustration
    c. Play skills increases
    d. All of the above

12. Which of the following is true about 3 year olds?
    a. They talk and ask questions constantly
    b. Imitating adults is common
    c. They are less fearful of strangers
    d. All of the above

13. Which of the following is a development task of a child in school age?
    a. Developing a conscience and morals
    b. Learning gender differences
    c. Performing self care
    d. Learning to play with others

14. Which of the following occurs in the school age group?
    a. They can sing simple songs
    b. Rivalry with siblings is common
    c. They are concerned about being well liked
    d. They enjoy playing dress up 15. School age is between ……….
    a. 1 to 3
    b. 3 to 6
    c. 6 to 9
    d. 10 to 12

16. Which of the following is a development task for a child in the late childhood stage?
    a. Becoming independent of adults
    b. Developing and keeping friendships with peers
    c. Learning how to study
    d. All of the above

17. Which of the following occurs in late childhood?
    a. Friends share information about sex
    b. Parent and children may be uncomfortable discussing sex with each other
    c. Peer groups are the center of activities
    d. All of the above

18. Which of the following is a development task in the adolescence stage?

a. Preparing for marriage and family

b. Developing moral and ethical behavior

c. Learning how to study

d. Understanding the social role of one's sex

19. ....marks the beginning of puberty in girls

a. Pubic hair

b. Menarche

c. Budding breast

d. Nocturnal emissions

20. Which of the following is a development task in young adulthood?

a. Coping with partner's death

b. Developing new friends

c. Selecting a partner

d. Having grown parents

21. People marry for which of the following reasons?

a. Love

b. Emotional security

c. Wanting a family

d. All of the above

22. Which of the following is a developmental task in middle adulthood?

a. Adjusting to physical changes

b. Developing a satisfactory sex life

c. Becoming a parent

d. Choosing a career

23. Menopause occurs between the age of ....

a. 30 to 45

b. 45 to 55

c. 55 to 65

d. 65 to 70

24. Which of the following is a developmental task in late adulthood?

a. Adjusting to decreased strength

b. Adjusting to loss of health

c. Preparing for ones death

d. All of the above

25. Late adulthood is between ....

a. 40 to 50 years

b. 40 to 65 years

c. 50 to 70 years

d.   65 years and older

Section 11

Care of the older person

1. Which of the following is true about old age?
   a. Chronic illness is common in older persons
   b. Disability increases
   c. Income may reduce
   d. All of the above
2. Which of the following is NOT true about aging
   a. Aging means illness
   b. Some old people are crabby
   c. They may process information slowly
   d. They are at risk of health problems
3. Which of the following is a physical reminder of old age?
   a. Retirement
   b. Gray hair
   c. Reduced income
   d. Children leaving home
4. Which of the following prevents loneliness?
   a. Hobbies
   b. Religious and community events
   c. Family times
   d. All of the above
5. Which of the following occurs in the integumentary system of an old person?
   a. The skin's blood vessels become more thick
   b. There is decreased secretion of oil
   c. Sweat increases
   d. All of the above
6. Which of the following must be done when taking care of an older person?
   a. Bath daily to ensure hygiene
   b. Use antiseptic soap always
   c. Use lotion and creams
   d. Use deodorant always
7. Which of the following is true about the nervous system of older people?
   a. There is increased blood flow to the brain
   b. Increased memory
   c. Brain tissue may atrophy
   d. Reflexes increase
8. When a patient complains of cold feet, which of the following should be done?
   a. Provide heating pads
   b. Provide hot water bottles

c. Provide socks

d. Massage feet

9. Which of the following occurs in the circulatory system as old age approaches?

    a. Heart walls thickens

    b. Number of red blood cells increases

    c. Heart valves thin out

    d. Arteries widen

10. Which of the following will help to prevent bone loss and loss of muscle strength?

    a. Exercise

    b. Engaging in activities

    c. Good diet

    d. All of the above

11. Which of the following changes occur in the senses of older people?

    a. Bitter and sour taste are lost first

    b. Eyelids thin

    c. There is increased tear secretion

    d. The pupil becomes larger

12. Which of the following occurs in the digestive system?

    a. More saliva is produced

    b. Increased appetite

    c. Digestive juice increases

    d. Peristalsis decreases

13. Which of the following is true about the urinary system of older persons?

    a. The kidneys shrink

    b. The kidney function increases

    c. Bladder size increases

    d. All of the above

14. Which of the following can be done to aid hearing loss within the home?

    a. Install lights in closets and stairways

    b. Install automatic garage door opener

    c. Install doorbells than can be heard throughout the house

    d. Remove scatter or throw rugs

15. Continuing care retirement communities offer which of the following services?

    a. Transportation

    b. Personal assistance

    c. Housekeeping

    d.   All of the above

Section 12

Safety

1. .... is the state of being aware of one's setting and being unable to react or respond to people. a. Coma
   b. Confusion
   c. Shock
   d. Disorientation
2. Which of the following people are at risk of accident?
   a. Children
   b. Old people
   c. People with vision loss
   d. All of the above
3. ......means loss of muscle function, sensation or both in the leg
   a. Hemiplegia
   b. Quadriplegia
   c. Paraplegia
   d. None of the above
4. Which of the following safety measure should be taken for infants and children?
   a. Leave children near open windows
   b. Store knives in upper cabinets
   c. Leave babies in walkers with wheels
   d. Leave children with toys and car strollers
5. Which of the following should be done to ensure safety?
   a. Do not use a crib with loose part
   b. Keep electrical appliances away from sinks
   c. Remove loops from blinds
   d. All of the above
6. When children are in the car, ...
   a. Ensure the windows are down when leaving them alone
   b. Let them play in the car
   c. Show them how to find and use the emergency trunk release mechanism
   d. Show them how to start the car
7. When children are in water areas, ...
   a. Have a phone by the pool

b. Keep diapers pail locked

c. Be aware of small bodies of water that can present danger

d. All of the above

8. Which of the following information is written on the ID bracelets?

a. The person's room number

b. The person's address

c. The person's religion

d. All of the above

9. ………involves the epidermis

a. Superficial burn

b. Partial thickness burn

c. Second degree burn

d. Full thickness burn

10. In ………. The nerve endings are destroyed

a. Superficial burn

b. Third degree burn

c. Fourth degree burn

d. Second degree burn

11. Which of the following is a characteristic of 3rd degree burn?

a. The skin appears deep red

b. The skin is painful to touch

c. The skin has black patches

d. There may be mild swelling

12. In a 68□C, it takes …….. for a third degree burn to occur

a. 5 minutes

b. 3 minutes

c. 1 minute

d. 1 second

13. Which of the following is a poison?

a. Soap

b. Paint

c. Wild mushrooms

d. All of the above

14. Which of the following is a sign and symptom of lead poisoning in children?

a. Memory problems

b. Diabetes

c. Dyspnea

d. All of the above

15. Lead is found in ………

a. Alcohol

b. Plastics

c. Shampoos

d. Mouthwash

16. Which of the following is a characteristic of carbon monoxide poisoning?
    a. It is colorless
    b. It has a bad odor
    c. It is produced from dust
    d. All of the above

17. Which of the following is a sign of carbon monoxide poisoning?
    a. Constipation
    b. Diarrhea
    c. Vomiting
    d. Pallor

18. Which of the following is done to prevent suffocation?
    a. Use pillows to position infants
    b. Use pillow to prevent infants from falling off the bed
    c. Tie large plastic bags and garment bags in knots
    d. All of the above

19. Which of the following is a way of relieving choking in the infant
    a. Give up to 5 forceful back slaps with the heel of your hand
    b. Press the stomach forcefully
    c. Give abdominal thrust
    d. All of the above

20. Which of the following should be done to prevent equipment accidents?
    a. Do not cover electrical cords with rugs
    b. Do not use power strips for care equipment
    c. Do not put finger into an electrical outlet
    d. All of the above

Section 13

Preventing falls

1. Which of the following is true according to the center for disease control and prevention?
   a. Falls are the main cause of injury related deaths in older adults
   b. Falls result disability
   c. Over one third of adults 65 years or older fall each year
   d. All of the above

2. Which of the following causes falls?
   a. Bright lighting
   b. Out of place furniture
   c. Lighted hallways

d. Dry floor

3. Most falls occur in the ………
   a. Morning
   b. Afternoon
   c. Night
   d. Daylight

4. Which of the following increases the risk of falls
   a. Vision problems
   b. Unsteadiness
   c. Frequent urination
   d. All of the above

5. To reduce falls, ensure ……….
   a. Bathrooms should have grab bars
   b. Bedpan or urinal should be out of reach
   c. Tubs should have slippery surfaces
   d. Skid wax should be used on hardwood

6. Which of the following is true about bed rails?
   a. It can cause entrapment
   b. Drop side cribs should be used
   c. All old persons must use rails
   d. All of the above

7. Grab bars are in the ……….
   a. Hallway
   b. Bathroom
   c. Rooms
   d. Dining rooms

8. Which of the following should be noted when using transfer or gait belts?
   a. It should be applied over the skin
   b. Excess straps should be left dangling
   c. Breast must not be caught under the skin
   d. It must be positioned over the person's spine

9. Which of the following should be done when a fall is about to occur or has occurred?
   a. Prevent the fall
   b. Help the person up
   c. Ease the person to the floor
   d. All of the above

10. Which of the following should be done when a bariatric person starts to fall?
    a. Try to protect the person's head
    b. Ease the person to the floor
    c. Let the person's buttocks rest on your leg
d.   Help the person back up

Section 14

Restraint alternatives and safe restraint use

1. ....is any drug used for discipline or convenience and not required to treat medical symptoms
   a. Physical restraint
   b. Chemical restraint
   c. Psychological restraint
   d. Medical restraint
2. Which of the following is a risk of restraint use?
   a. Anger
   b. Constipation
   c. Dehydration
   d. All of the above
3. Restraints should be used to ....
   a. Discipline
   b. Punish
   c. Prevent the patient from harm
   d. Penalize
4. Which of the following is an alternative to restraint use?
   a. Providing a calm environment
   b. Not answering the signal light immediately
   c. Not meeting elimination needs
   d. Keeping bedpans away from the patient
5. .... is a device that limits freedom of movement but is used to promote independence or comfort a. Restraint
   b. Enabler
   c. Enhancer
   d. Comforter
6. Restraints can cause which of the following?
   a. Low self esteem
   b. Death
   c. Fractures
   d. All of the above

7. Center for Medicare and Medicaid services requires the reporting of any death that occurs ……….
    a. While a person was in restraint
    b. Within 8 days after restraint was removed
    c. Within 2 weeks after restraint was removed
    d. Within 1 month after which restraint was removed

8. When using restraint which of the following should be noted?
    a. It should be used as first resort
    b. The most restrictive method should be used
    c. Informed consent is required
    d. A nurse must order the restraint

9. Which of the following should be done when a patient is restrained?
    a. Observe the person at most twice in a day
    b. Ensure the restraint is tight
    c. Apply restraint with enough help to protect the person from injury
    d. All of the above

10. When applying restraints, …………
    a. Use it to position the person on a toilet
    b. Use it to position a person on furniture that does not allow for correct application
    c. Position the person alignment
    d. Criss-cross straps in the back

11. Which of the following precautions should be taken when applying restraints?
    a. Apply a belt restraint at a 45 degree angle over the thighs
    b. Make sure the straps are tight
    c. Secure the restraints to the bed rails
    d. All of the above

12. After applying the restraints, …………
    a. Use back cushion when a person is restrained in a chair
    b. Monitor persons in the supine position constantly
    c. Check the person every one hour
    d. Cover the person with a blanket

13. When restraints are released, which of the following needs must be met?
    a. Food needs
    b. Hygiene needs
    c. Elimination needs
    d. All of the above

14. Which of the following should be reported and recorded when observing a person in restraint?
    a. The person's vital sign
    b. Conditions of the limb

c. The type of restraint applied

d. All of the above

15. Leather restraints are applied on the ....

    a. Chest

    b. Hands

    c. Ankles

    d. Breast

16. ....is used when a person is at risk for pulling out tubes used for life saving

treatment

    a. Jacket restraints

    b. Wrist restraints

    c. Belt restraints

    d. Leather restraints

17. A belt restraint is used for which of the following?

    a. To prevent falls from bed or chair

    b. They prevent finger use

    c. To prevent pulling at devices used to monitor vital signs

    d. All of the above

18. Which of the following is true about vest restraints?

    a. They are used to prevent injuries from falls

    b. The person will be able to turn and get out of bed without help

    c. It should be applied under the garment

    d. All of the above

19. Restraints should not be used if the person has ....

    a. Colostomy

    b. Gastrostomy tube

    c. Incisions

    d. All of the above

20. When using a mitt restraint, ensure ....

    a. The person is strapped at 90 degrees angle

    b. The person's hands are clean

    c. Zippers are closed

    d. The vest is free of wrinkles

Section 15

Preventing infection

1. Which of the following are at risk of infection?
   a. Infants
   b. Older persons
   c. Disabled persons
   d. All of the above
2. Microbes can be found in the ………
   a. Mouth
   b. Nose
   c. Stomach
   d. All of the above
3. …………are one celled organisms that multiply rapidly and are often called germs
   a. Bacteria
   b. Fungi
   c. Protozoa
   d. Virus
4. ……….are plant like organisms that live on other plants or animals
   a. Virus
   b. Fungi
   c. Bacteria
   d. None of the above
5. ………..causes diseases such as cold, herpes and hepatitis
   a. Rickettsiae
   b. Protozoa
   c. Viruses
   d. Fungi
6. Rickettsiae causes……….
   a. Immunodeficiency syndrome
   b. Rocky mountain spotted fever
   c. Herpes
   d. Common cold
7. Which of the following is needed for microbes to live and grow?
   a. Water
   b. Heat
   c. Light
   d. All of the above
8. E.coli is normally found in the ………..
   a. Colon
   b. Liver
   c. Brain
   d. Lungs

9. Which of the following is true about Methicillin resistant Staphylococcus aureus?
   a. It is normally found in the colon
   b. It is resistant to antibiotics often used for Staph infections
   c. It is transmitted through toilet seats
   d. All of the above

10. Which of the following is true about Vancomycin resistant Enterococci
    a. It can cause pneumonia
    b. It is normally found in the lungs
    c. It can cause urinary tract
    d. It is normally found in the nose

11. Which of the following is a sign and symptom of infection?
    a. Confusion
    b. Nausea
    c. Vomiting
    d. All of the above

12. A ……..is a carrier that transmits disease
    a. Pathogen
    b. Vector
    c. Carrier
    d. Source

13. ………. Carries rabies
    a. Dogs
    b. Mosquitoes
    c. Ticks
    d. Mites

14. A pathogen enters the body through …………
    a. Portal of exit
    b. Portal of entry
    c. Susceptible host
    d. Reservoir

15. Which of the following is a common site for healthcare-associated infection?
    a. The bloodstream
    b. Wounds
    c. The urinary system
    d. All of the above

16. ………is the process of becoming unclean
    a. Sterilization
    b. Contamination
    c. Infection
    d. Vaccination

17. Which of the following is a common aseptic practice?

a. Brush teeth once in a while

b. Eat raw fruits often

c. Washing of hands after sneezing

d. Bathe once a week

18. To prevent microbes in the home, ………..

a. Flush toilet after each use

b. Remove and dispose hair from the sink

c. Wipe out water spills

d. All of the above

19. Which of the following procedures should be followed when washing your hands?

a. Use hot water

b. Do not touch inside the sink

c. Use your uniform to dry your hands

d. All of the above

20. Which of the following procedures should be followed when cleaning?

a. Wear personal protective equipment

b. Work from dirty to clean areas

c. Use hot water to remove organic matter

d. All of the above

21. ………..is the process of destroying pathogens

a. Sterilization

b. Cleaning

c. Disinfection

d. Vaccination

22. Which of the following is true about disinfection?

a. It destroys all non pathogens and pathogens

b. Very high temperatures are used

c. Spores are not destroyed

d. It can be done through radiation

23. Which of the following should be done to control portals of exit?

a. Cover your nose and mouth when coughing or sneezing

b. Keep tables and other surfaces clean

c. Keep bottles and fluid containers tightly capped

d. Use leak proof plastic bags for solid tissues

24. Which of the following is a common communicable childhood disease?

a. Chickenpox

b. Measles

c. Scarlet fever

d. All of the above

25. Scarlet fever is transmitted through ……….

a. Contact with urine of the infected person

b. Handshake

c. Sharing of plates and cups

d. Contact with nasal secretion

26. Which of the following precautions should be followed to prevent infection?

a. Do not wear fake nails if you have contact with persons at risk for infection

b. Wash gloves for re-use

c. Re-use gowns for contact with the same person

d. All of the above

27. Which of the following is true about airborne infection isolation rooms?

a. It has more than one occupant

b. The room door is kept closed except when a person enters or leaves the room

c. Treatments are carried out outside the AIIR room

d. All of the above

28. Which of the following is a precaution that should be taken when entering and leaving the isolation room?

a. Collect items needed in bits before entering the room

b. Shake linens vigorously when making beds

c. Use paper towels to handle contaminated items

d. Use your bare hands to open and close the door of the room

29. Which of the following should be done when handling contaminated laundry?

a. Wear gloves

b. Carry contaminated laundry from the patient room to the nurse station for bagging

c. Place wet contaminated laundry on the floor

d. All of the above

30. Which of the following is an appropriate way of managing waste items?

a. Flush needles down the toilet

b. Throw syringes into the garbage

c. Put needles in the recycle container

d. Store syringes in a puncture resistant container

Section 16

Body mechanics

1. Which of the following is a function of the musculo-skeletal system?

a. It gives the body shape

b. It protects the internal organs

c. It lets the body move

d. All of the above

2. Which of the following is a function of long bones?

   a. They bear the weight of the body

   b. They protect the internal organ

   c. They allow ease of movement

   d. They protect the spinal column

3. Which of the following is true about hinge joints?

   a. It is immovable

   b. It allows movement in all directions

   c. It allows movement in one direction

   d. It allows turning from side to side

4. Involuntary muscles are found in the …….

   a. Stomach

   b. Arms

   c. Legs

   d. All of the above

5. The strongest muscles of the body are located in the ………

   a. Fingers

   b. Shoulders

   c. Stomach

   d. Blood vessels

6. Which of the following is a rule for body mechanics?

   a. Bend your back

   b. Pull heavy objects

   c. Do not lean over a person to give care

   d. Lift objects above your shoulders to maintain balance

7. Which of the following is true about work related musculo-skeletal disorder?

   a. The arms and back are often affected

   b. They are developed slowly

   c. Stiff joints may occur

   d. All of the above

8. Which of the following is a sign of back injury?

   a. Decreased mobility

   b. Pain when trying to assume a normal posture

   c. Poor physical conditions

   d. All of the above

9. ……….is a semi sitting position

   a. Fowler's position

   b. Supine position

c. Prone position

d. Lateral position

10. Which of the following is true about supine position?

    a. The person lies on one side or the other

    b. The head of the bed is raised between 45 and 60 degrees

    c. It is the back lying position

    d. It is a semi prone side position

Section 17

Safely moving and transferring the person

1. To safely move or transfer a person, the health team should determine ....

    a. The person's dependence level

    b. The amount of assistance needed

    c. What procedure to use

    d. All of the above

2. Which of the following should be done when moving or transferring a person?

    a. Don't ask for help

    b. Move the person carefully

    c. Place the person's face against a pillow

    d. All of the above

3. When using manual lifting, which of the following should be done?

    a. Move the person away from you

    b. Lower the person bending your back

    c. Avoid jerking movement

    d. Twist and turn when lifting a person

4. When transporting the person and equipment, ...

    a. Pull the equipment

    b. Use an upright posture

    c. Keep the load away from the body

    d. All of the above

5. Which of the following is true about code 1 level of dependence?

    a. The person can walk without help

    b. The staff needs to look after the person

    c. The person cannot help the transfer

    d. The person can still bear some weight

6. Which of the following is true about code 4 level of dependence?

    a. The person is lifted with a full sling mechanical lift

    b. The person needs some help moving legs

c. Sling boards are useful for transfers to and from beds

d. Mechanical assistance is not normally required

7. Which of the following should be done when moving a person with dementia?

    a. Force the person to move

    b. Help the person alone

    c. Use a calm voice

    d. Proceed quickly to avoid distraction

8. A mechanical lift should be used to help lift a person ………

    a. On code 4 with total dependence

    b. On Code 0 level of dependence

    c. On code 2 level of dependence

    d. On code 1 level of dependence

9. …….. is when the skin sticks to a surface while muscle slide in the direction the body is moving a. Tearing

    b. Shearing

    c. Friction

    d. Shredding

10. Which of the following precautions should be followed when turning a person?

    a. Turn the person away from you with the far bed rail down

    b. Do not logroll older persons

    c. Use pillows to support the person in the side lying position

    d. All of the above

11. Which of the following should be done when logrolling a person?

    a. Ensure the bed is in a fowler's position

    b. It is used for person's with spinal cord injuries

    c. It should not be used for older patients

    d. All of the above

12. Which of the following precautions should be followed before and after putting a patient in a dangling position? a. Only one staff member is needed

    b. It should be done for persons who need extensive assistance

    c. Raise the head of the bed to a sitting position

    d. Leave the person alone to promote independence

13. When transferring a person to a wheelchair,………

    a. Lower the bed to its lowest positions

    b. Put the persons arm around your neck

    c. Unlock the wheelchair wheels

    d. All of the above

14. Which of the following should be done when transferring from wheelchair to the bed?

    a. Transfer from the weak side

    b. Lock the wheelchair wheels

    c.   Unlock the bed wheels

    d.   Position the weak side on the near the bed

15. ....are used for normal transfers

    a.   Standard full swing

    b.   Toileting sling

    c.   Bathing sling

    d.   Extended sling

16. ....are used for persons with extra large thighs

    a.   Standard full swing

    b.   Extra large swing

    c.   Extended length swing

    d.   Extra full swing

17. In ....the sling is open at the bottom

    a.   Bathing sling

    b.   Toileting sling

    c.   Open and close sling

    d.   Extra full swing

18. A sling is contaminated if ....

    a.   It has any visible sign of blood

    b.   It is used on a person's bare skin

    c.   It is used to bathe a person

    d.   All of the above

19. If a person weighs more than 200 pounds which of the following is recommended when moving a person to a stretcher? a. Use a lateral sliding aid and 1 staff member

    b.   A friction reducing device and 1 staff member

    c.   A mechanical lateral transfer device with in built slide board

    d.   All of the above

20. Which of the following should be done when repositioning a person on the wheelchair?

    a.   Lock the wheels

    b.   Pull the person from behind the chair

    c.   Unlock the wheels of the chair

d.   Carry the person from the bed to the chair

Section 18

The person's unit

  1. Most healthy people are comfortable when the temperature is ....

a. 68□F to 74□F

b. 40□F to 50□F

c. 30□F to 50□F

d. 50□F to 100□F

2. Which of the following is true about less active persons?

a. They need to dress lightly

b. The like cool areas

c. They like warm room temperatures

d. All of the above

3. Which of the following protects older persons from drafts?

a. Providing them with warm blankets

b. Moving them from drafty areas

c. Giving them lap robes

d. All of the above

4. Which of the following is an OBRA requirement?

a. Rooms should have direct access to exit corridor

b. The corridor should have functioning call systems

c. Rooms should be cleaned twice daily

d. Each room should have a television

5. Which of the following should be done to reduce odors?

a. Empty urinals promptly

b. Ensure toilets are flushed

c. Clean persons who are wet or soiled from urine

d. All of the above

6. According to CMS, a comfortable sound level should ………

a. Interfere slightly with a person's hearing

b. Promote privacy

c. Increase patient's sleep opportunity

d. All of the above

7. Which of the following can be used to reduce noise?

a. Do not use metal equipments

b. Use plastic dishes

c. Do not talk loudly

d. Do not repair equipments when residents are sleeping 8. Which of the following can cause falls?

a. Glares

b. Dull lighting

c. Shadows

d. All of the above

9. In manual beds …….. raises or lowers the head of the bed

a. Right crank

b. Left crank

c. Center crank

d. Matching crank

10. The .... of the manual bed adjusts the knee portion

    a. Right crank

    b. Center crank

    c. Left crank

    d. Matching crank

11. In the ....position the head of the bed is raised 30 degrees and the knee is raised at 15 degrees

    a. Fowler's position

    b. Trendelenburg's position

    c. Semi fowler's position

    d. High fowler's position

12. Which of the following is true about the Trendelenburg's position?

    a. The doctor orders the position

    b. The head of the bed is raised 60 degrees

    c. It is used after a spinal cord injury

    d. All of the above

13. In ....the head of the bed is raised and the foot of the bed is lowered

    a. High fowler

    b. Fowler's position

    c. Reverse Trendelenburg's position

    d. Trendelenburg's position

14. Which of the following is true about the flat bed position?

    a. It is used after cervical traction surgery

    b. It is ordered by a doctor

    c. The bed frame s tilted

    d. All of the above

15. Which of the following are at risk of entrapment?

    a. Older residents

    b. Confused residents

    c. Disoriented residents

    d. All of the above

16. Which of the following is a feature of the bariatric beds?

    a. It can be converted to a chair

    b. It has built on scale

    c. It can be used as a stretcher

    d. All of the above

17. Which of the following can be placed on the bedside stand?

    a. Bedpans

    b. Urinals

    c. Kidney basin

d. Soiled linen

18. The call system should be placed in which of locations in the facility?
    a. The bathroom
    b. The facility entrance
    c. The corridor
    d. The emergency exit

19. The signal light should be placed……..
    a. Within the person's reach
    b. At the person's weak side
    c. By the door
    d. All of the above

20. Which of the following should be done when maintaining a person's unit?
    a. Move furniture around to allow space
    b. Straighten beds and linens
    c. Ensure very bright lights are in the room
    d. All of the above

Section 19

Bed making

1. A …….. bed is not in use
    a. Closed bed
    b. Open bed
    c. Occupied bed
    d. Surgical bed

2. Closed beds are made for ……..
    a. Residents who are in bed throughout the day
    b. Residents who are up throughout the day
    c. Persons who arrive in ambulance
    d. Persons who are already lying in it

3. …….. is made for persons who arrive by ambulance
    a. Ambulance bed
    b. Emergency bed
    c. Surgical bed
    d. Open bed

4. When handling linens,……..
    a. Hold them close to yourself
    b. Shake them

    c.   Place them on a clean surface

    d.   All of the above

5. Which of the following precautions should be followed when handling linens?

    a.   Use extra linen in another resident's room

    b.   Put dirty linen on the floor

    c.   Collect linens in the order of use

    d.   Always take extra linen to a person's room

6. When changing linen,.........

    a.   Change wet linens immediately

    b.   Re-use if it is wrinkled

    c.   Roll each piece towards you when removing

    d.   Remove the dirty linens all together at once

7. Which of the following is a function of the cotton drawsheet?

    a.   It protects the mattress from dampness

    b.   It beautifies the bed

    c.   It helps keep the bottom linen clean

    d.   It helps to straighten wrinkles on the bed

8. Which of the following is true about plastic covered mattress?

    a.   It reduces heat retention

    b.   It retains heat

    c.   It absorbs moisture

    d.   All of the above

9. Which of the following is a rule for bedmaking?

    a.   Use extra linen for another person

    b.   Do not use torn linen

    c.   Hold linen close to you

    d.   Place waterproof drawsheet on the top against the person's body 10.
Which of the following is a guideline for children's crib?

    a.   Use soft mattress

    b.   Antique crib must be approved by the nursing assistant

    c.   The space between the crib slats should not be more than 10 inches

    d.   The mattress must fit the crib

11. The mattress in a crib should be at least .... inches lower than the top of the crib side

    a.   2

    b.   5

    c.   10

    d.   26

12. Which of the following precautions should be considered when making a crib?

    a.   Use sheets for king size bed

    b.   Bumper pads should not be used

c. End panels should have cut outs

d. Place pillow towards the edge of the crib

13. Which of the following must be done if bumper pads are used in cribs?

a. It must cover the entire inside of the crib

b. It must fit snugly against the slats

c. At least 6 ties or snaps should be in place

d. All of the above

14. Open beds are made for ……….

a. Person's who are getting ready for bed

b. Residents who are up for most of the day

c. Persons who are using portable tubs

d. Person's who go by stretcher to treatment or therapy

15. Which of the following should be done when making surgical beds?

a. Place the linen on a clean surface

b. Remove the signal light

c. Raise the bed for body mechanics

d. All of the above

Section 20

Personal hygiene

1. The crown of the tooth is covered by ……..

a. Enamel

b. Gum

c. Dentin

d. Neck

2. Which of the following is true about the epidermis?

a. It has living cells

b. It has dead cells

c. It has few nerve endings

d. All of the above

3. Which of the following is true about the dermis?

a. It has dead cells

b. It has blood vessels in it

c. It is made up of dead cells

d. None of the above

4. Which of the following is a function of the skin?

a. It stores fat and water

b. It provides the body's protective covering

c. It prevent microbes from entering the body

d. All of the above

5. AM care includes which of the following?

   a. Assisting with elimination

   b. Cleaning incontinent persons

   c. Making beds and straightening units

   d. All of the above

6. ....is given after breakfast

   a. AM care

   b. Morning care

   c. Afternoon care

   d. Evening care

7. Which of the following is done in evening care?

   a. Assisting with range of motion exercise

   b. Positioning for breakfast

   c. Helping persons change into sleepwear

   d. Assisting with ambulation

8. ....is a thin film that sticks to the teeth, it contains saliva and microbes

   a. Tartar

   b. Pyorrhea

   c. Plague

   d. Dental carries

9. Tartar causes which of the following?

   a. Periodontal disease

   b. Swollen gum

   c. Tooth loss

   d. All of the above

10. Baby bottle tooth decay is common in the ....

    a. Upper front teeth

    b. Lower back teeth

    c. Gum

    d. Upper back teeth

11. Which of the following can be done to prevent baby bottle tooth decay?

    a. Wipe the baby's gum with clean damp gauze pad washcloth

    b. Bottles should be finished before bed time

    c. Do not dip a pacifier in sugar or honey

    d. All of the above

12. If done once a day, ...is the best time to floss

    a. Morning

    b. After lunch

c. Before bed time

d. After breakfast

13. To prevent aspiration in an unconscious person...........
    a. Use small amount of fluid to clean the mouth
    b. Position the person lying flat
    c. Clean dentures in the mouth
    d. Use your fingers for hard to reach areas

14. Which of the following is true about dentures
    a. They should be wrapped in a napkin
    b. Store in a cold denture solution
    c. Use toothpaste to clean them
    d. Place them in hot water to remove germs

15. Which of the following rules should be followed when giving baths
    a. Close doors and windows
    b. Cover the person for warmth
    c. Wash from the cleanest to the dirtiest area
    d. All of the above

16. .... Is used to mask and control body odors
    a. Antiperspirants
    b. Powders
    c. Deodorants
    d. Soap

17. Which of the following procedures should be followed about skin care?
    a. Older patients should have their bath daily with soap to reduce risk of infection
    b. Provide for warmth
    c. Use bath oil to reduce dry skin
    d. Deodorants can be used to replace bathing

18. Which of the following person's decide when to give a resident a bath?
    a. The nurse
    b. The nursing assistant
    c. The resident
    d. The doctor

19. Which of the following should be done during and after bathing?
    a. Use hot water for bath
    b. Sprinkle powder onto the person
    c. Apply the powder in a thin
    d. All of the above

20. Bed baths are usually given to which of the following persons?
    a. Unconscious persons
    b. Paralyzed persons
    c. Persons weak from illness

d. All of the above

21. Which of the following procedures should be followed when giving a tub bath?
    a. Do not leave weak persons unattended to
    b. Get the person out of the tub before draining the tub
    c. It should not last for more than 60 minutes
    d. Use bath oils always

22. Which of the following rules should be observed when giving back massage?
    a. It should not exceed 30 minutes
    b. Massage reddened bony areas slightly
    c. Use lotion to reduce friction
    d. All of the above

23. Perineal care is important for which of the following persons?
    a. Persons with urinary catheters
    b. Persons menstruating
    c. Uncircumcised persons
    d. All of the above

24. Which of the following should be done when giving perineal care?
    a. Use cotton balls to clean
    b. Clean from the dirtiest to the cleanest area
    c. Use hot water to clean
    d. All of the above

25. Which of the following should be reported if observed while cleaning
    a. Bleeding
    b. Unusual odors
    c. Signs of skin breakdown
    d. All of the above

Section 21

Grooming

1. ....means hair loss
    a. Alopecia
    b. Hirsutism
    c. Dandruff
    d. Pediculosis

2. Which of the following is a cause of alopecia?
    a. Stress

b. Skin disease

c. Pregnancy

d. All of the above

3. ....is excessive body hair

a. Pediculosis

b. Hirsutism

c. Alopecia

d. None of the above

4. Which of the following is true about lice?

a. They hatch in 1 day

b. They feed on hair

c. They bite the scalp

d. They are black in color

5. ....is the infestation of the pubic hair with lice

a. Pediculosis pubis

b. Pediculosis capitis

c. Pediculosis infestation

d. Pediculosis corporis

6. Lice can be spread through ....

a. Clothing

b. Beds

c. Sexual contact

d. All of the above

7. Which of the following can be done to prevent lice spreading?

a. Wash cloths with hot water

b. Sweep the entire room

c. Eat fruits and raw vegetables

d. All of the above

8. Scabies is caused by ....

a. Lice

b. Female mite

c. Roaches

d. Mosquitoes

9. Which of the following is a common site of scabies?

a. Between fingers

b. Face

c. Back of ears

d. Scalp

10. Which of the following is true about scabies?

a. It is highly contagious

b. Children are more at risk

c. It hatches within 4 days

d. All of the above

11. Which of the following should be done when brushing and combing hair?
    a. Cut away matted hair while combing
    b. Choose how to style the hair
    c. Use a wide tooth comb for curly hair
    d. All of the above

12. Which of the following is a shampoo method?
    a. Shampoo at the sink
    b. Shampoo in bed
    c. Shampoo on a stretcher
    d. All of the above

13. People with limited range of motion in their necks should be shampooed ………
    a. At the sink
    b. On a stretcher
    c. On the bed
    d. All of the above

14. Safety razors should be used for ………
    a. Elderly persons
    b. Persons taking anticoagulants
    c. Young patients
    d. Patients with healing problems

15. Which of the following should be noted before and during shaving?
    a. Soften the skin
    b. Shave against the direction of the hair growth
    c. Move razor in small circles while shaving
    d. All of the above

16. ………is a common cause of poor circulation in the foot?
    a. Constipation
    b. Diabetes
    c. Diarrhea
    d. Fever

17. Which of the following causes injuries on the foot?
    a. Stepping on sharp objects
    b. Poorly fitted shoes
    c. Being stepped on
    d. All of the above

18. Which of the following should be done when giving foot and nail care?
    a. Trim thick ingrown nails
    b. Put the person's feet inside hot water
    c. Apply lotion after trimming
    d. Soak the person's feet for 1 hour

19. Which of the following should be done when dressing and undressing for a resident?
    a. Choose the person's outfit
    b. Stack clothes in order they are out on
    c. Remove cloth from the weak or affected side first
    d. Help the patient as much as possible to speed up time
20. Which of the following should be done when changing hospital gowns?
    a. If patient has paralysis, put the clean gown on the strong arm first and then the weak hand
    b. Disconnect the IV set up to aid removal of dress
    c. In case the patient has injury, remove the gown from the strong arm first
    d. All of the above

Section 22

Urinary elimination

1. Urine is formed in the ....
    a. Bladder
    b. Kidney
    c. Urethra
    d. Ureter
2. The urinary system does which of the following?
    a. Remove carbon dioxide
    b. Removes solid waste
    c. Removes waste from the blood
    d. All of the above
3. A healthy adult produces about .... of urine a day
    a. 500ml
    b. 1500ml
    c. 3000ml
    d. 4500ml
4. Which of the following factors affect urine production?
    a. Age
    b. Disease
    c. Body temperature
    d. All of the above
5. Which of the following should be done if a person cannot start the stream of urine?
    a. Run water in the sink

    b. Stand in the toilet

    c. Pat the person's back

    d. Give the person more fluid 6. Normal urine color is ....

a. Pale yellow

b. Red

c. Tea

d. Brown

7. Which of the following causes nocturia?

    a. Urinary tract disease

    b. Shock

    c. Kidney disease

    d. Trauma

8. Which of the following causes urinary incontinence?

    a. Aging

    b. Urinary tract infection

    c. Trauma

    d. All of the above

9. Fracture pans are used by ....

    b. Persons with casts

    c. Persons in traction

    d. After a hip fracture

    e. All of the above

10. Men use ...... to void

    a. Bariatric bedpan

    b. Urinal

    c. Standard bedpan

    d. Fracture pan

11. ....is when urine leaks during exercise and certain movements that cause pressure on the bladder a. Stress incontinence

    b. Mixed incontinence

    c. Urge incontinence

    d. Reflex incontinence

12. Which of the following is a cause of urge incontinence?

    a. Late pregnancy

    b. Obesity

    c. Urinary urgency

    d. Menopause

13. Which of the following causes overflow incontinence?

    a. Sneezing

    b. Lifting

    c. Urinary urgency

    d. Diabetes

14. In …….. the person has bladder control but cannot us the toilet in time
    a. Overflow incontinence
    b. Functional incontinence
    c. Mixed incontinence
    d. Urge incontinence
15. Which of the following is a cause of transient incontinence?
    a. Urinary tract infection
    b. Bladder cancer
    c. Nervous system disorder
    d. Alzheimer's disease
16. Which of the following can be done to prevent urinary tract infection?
    a. Have the person wear cotton underwear
    b. Promote fluid intake
    c. Keep the perineal area clean and dry
    d. All of the above
17. Which of the following is a cause of bedwetting?
    a. Anxiety
    b. Nervous system disorder
    c. Confusion
    d. Bladder cancer
18. Which of the following guideline should be followed when applying incontinence products?
    a. For men position the penis upwards
    b. Center the product in the perineal area
    c. Let the plastic backing touch the person's skin
    d. All of the above
19. A ………drains the bladder and then is removed
    a. Foley catheter
    b. Retention catheter
    c. Straight catheter
    d. Direct catheter
20. Catheters are used to ……….
    a. Collect sterile urine specimen
    b. Measure the amount of urine left in the bladder after the person voids
    c. Keep the bladder empty
    d. All of the above
21. Which of the following should be done when caring for persons with indwelling catheters?
    a. The person should not lie on the tubing
    b. Hang drainage bag on the bed rail
    c. Place the drainage bag on the floor when full
    d. Let the tubing loop below the drainage bag

22. Which of the following should be done when changing a drainage bag?
    a. Place the bag on the floor
    b. Hold the ends of the catheter carefully when cleaning it
    c. Wipe the end of the tubing with an antiseptic
    d. All of the above

23. Which of the following should be done when removing indwelling catheter?
    a. Remove the catheter with water in the balloon to reduce pain of removal
    b. Deflate the balloon
    c. Pierce the balloon with the syringe from any location on the balloon
    d. All of the above

24. Which is true about condom catheters?
    a. They are called external catheters
    b. Adhesive is used to secure the catheter
    c. They are not self adhesive
    d. All of the above

25. Which of the following can help persons with urinary inconsistence?
    a. Bladder retraining
    b. Prompted voiding
    c. Catheter clamping
    d. All of the above

Section 23

Bowel elimination

1. Which of the following affects bowel elimination?
   a. Privacy
   b. Age
   c. Diet
   d. All of the above

2. ....causes red colored stools
   a. Bleeding in the stomach
   b. Bleeding in the small intestine
   c. Bleeding in the lower colon
   d. Bleeding in the bladder

3. Which of the following can cause green stools?
   a. Beets
   b. Tomato juice
   c. Vegetables
   d. Bleeding the colon

4. Chyme becomes less fluid and more solid when it enters the ......
   a. Stomach
   b. Large intestine
   c. Small intestine
   d. Anus
5. Feces are stored in the .... until they are ready to be excreted
   a. Large intestine
   b. Rectum
   c. Anus
   d. Duodenum
6. Adult stools are usually ....
   a. Liquid like
   b. Greenish brown
   c. Shaped like rectum
   d. Like thick liquid
7. Which of the following should be documented in your report?
   a. Color of stool
   b. Amount
   c. Consistency
   d. All of the above
8. Which of the following promotes bowel elimination?
   a. High fiber food
   b. Lack of privacy
   c. Bread
   d. All of the above
9. Which of the following stimulates peristalsis?
   a. Cauliflower
   b. Radishes
   c. Cabbage
   d. All of the above
10. Which of the following is true about constipation?
   a. It is the passage of hard stool
   b. The person cannot have a bowel movement
   c. The rectum is infected
   d. The feces moves fast from the rectum
11. Which of the following is used to treat constipation?
   a. Stool softeners
   b. Laxatives
   c. Enemas
   d. All of the above
12. ....is the prolonged retention and buildup of feces in the rectum
   a. Constipation

b. Fecal incontinence

c. Fecal impaction

d. Feces blockage

13. Which of the following can cause fecal incontinence?

a. Diarrhea

b. Aging

c. Intestinal diseases

d. All of the above

14. Which of the following is a cause of flatulence?

a. Constipation

b. Diarrhea

c. Aging

d. Fecal impaction

15. ....is a solution of salt and water

a. Tap water enema

b. Saline enema

c. Soapsuds enema

d. Small volume enema

16. In small volume enema, the adult size contains about..........of solution

a. 120 ml

b. 300 ml

c. 500ml

d. 1000ml

17. Which of the following should be observed when giving enemas?

a. Give the solution quickly

b. Raise the enema bag 50 inches above the anus for adults

c. Lubricate the tip before insertion

d. All of the above

18. Oil retention enema has ....

a. Cottonseed oil

b. Mineral oil

c. Olive oil

d. All of the above

19. Which of the following is true about enema?

a. Tap water enema should be repeated slowly

b. Repeated soapsud enemas can damage the bowel

c. Use only about 10ml of castile soap or stronger

d. Only the nurse can order enema

20. ....is a surgically created opening between small intestine and the abdominal wall a. Ostomy

b. Colostomy

c. Ileostomy

d. Ostomy pouch

Section 24

Nutrition and fluids

1. A poor diet can cause ....
   a. Increased risk of infection
   b. Healing problems
   c. Chronic illness to become worse
   d. All of the above
2. ....pushes food into the esophagus
   a. Contraction of the pharynx
   b. Movement of the tongue
   c. The salivary glands
   d. Involuntary muscle contractions
3. The first part of the small intestine is called ......
   a. Ileum
   b. Jejunum
   c. Duodenum
   d. Villi
4. ....absorbs digested food into the capillaries
   a. Chyme
   b. Villi
   c. Gastric juice
   d. Bile
5. 1 gram of fat equals to ....
   a. 9 calories
   b. 4 calories
   c. 7 calories
   d. 1 calorie
6. USDA recommends that an adult should do at least which of the following?
   a. 2 hours and 30 minutes of vigorous exercise
   b. 1 hour of moderate exercise
   c. Physical activity at least 3 days a week
   d. All of the above

7. According to myplate servings women should have ……. Cups of dairy in a day
    a. 8
    b. 5
    c. 3
    d. 1
8. Which of the following is an example of vigorous exercise?
    a. Canoeing
    b. Aerobics
    c. Dancing
    d. Gardening
9. Which of the following can be done to help children eat vegetable and fruits?
    b. Offer dried fruit in place of candy
    c. Top cereal with berries
    d. Let children help shop for vegetables
    e. All of the above
10. Which of the following is an example of whole grains?
    a. White flour
    b. Oatmeal
    c. White bread
    d. White rice
11. Green bananas belong to which of the following group?
    a. Starchy vegetables
    b. Dark green vegetable
    c. Beans
    d. Red and orange vegetable
12. Vegetable gave which of the following benefits?
    a. May prevent birth defects
    b. May reduce the risk of bone loss
    c. May reduce the risk of developing kidney stones
    d. All of the above
13. Which of the following is true about protein food?
    a. Egg whites are high in cholesterol
    b. Liver is low in cholesterol
    c. Processed meats have added salt
    d. All of the above
14. Which of the following is true about oils?
    a. It is a food group
    b. Adult women are allowed 8 to 10 teaspoon of oil daily
    c. Oils from plants do not contain cholesterol
    d. Adult men are allowed 1 to 12 teaspoon of oil a day
15. Oils and solid fats have about ………calories in each tablespoon
    a. 3

b. 40

c. 100

d. 120

16. ....is the most important nutrients

a. Oil

b. Protein

c. Vitamins

d. Carbohydrates

17. Which of the following is not digested?

a. Fats

b. Protein

c. Fiber

d. Milk

18. ....aids blood clotting

a. Vitamin K

b. Vitamin E

c. Vitamin D

d. Vitamin A

19. Which of the following is a source of vitamin D?

a. Fish liver oil

b. Tomatoes

c. Green vegetables

d. Melons

20. Vitamin A does which of the following?

a. Helps protein metabolism

b. Aid the growth of healthy hair

c. Aids intestinal functions

d. All of the above

21. Which of the following affects eating and nutrition?

a. Culture

b. Religion

c. Finances

d. All of the above

22. Which of the following is an OBRA requirement for food served in nursing centers?

a. Each person must receive at least 4 meals a day

b. The food should be appetizing

c. It should be prepared by a professional chef

d. All food should be served hot 23. Which of the following is true?

a. Pork products can be served to Muslims

b. In Hinduism cows and cow products are allowed

c. Jews believe that food must be kosher

d. Seventh day Adventist allows caffeine but not alcohol 24. Which of the following is a mechanical soft food?

a. Whole wheat bread

b. Cooked fruits

c. Potatoes

d. Rice

e.

25. The body needs no more than ………. Sodium intake per day

a. 2300mg

b. 3000mg

c. 5000mg

d. 10000mg

26. Which of the following food is high in sodium?

a. Waffles

b. Relish

c. Cheese

d. All of the above

27. ………..is breathing fluid, food or an object into the lungs

a. Dysphagia

b. Aspiration

c. Dispiration

d. Hematuria

28. Which of the following is a sign and sympom of dysphagia?

a. Avoiding foods that needs chewing

b. Appetite decrease

c. The person eats solid slowly

d. All of the above

29. Which of the following can be done to prevent aspiration?

a. Give the person only liquid or semi liquid food

b. Help the person with meals and snacks

c. Avoid dairy products

d. Develop a meal plan

30. One pint is about ………

a. 30 ml

b. 50 ml

c. 100ml

d.   500ml

Nutritional support and IV therapy

1. ………is a common cause of poor nutrition
   a. Coma
   b. Dementia
   c. Dysphagia
   d. All of the above
2. ………is a feeding tube inserted through the nose into the stomach
   a. Naso-enteral tube
   b. Naso-gastric tube
   c. Gastrostomy tube
   d. Jejunostomy tube
3. Percutaneous endoscopic gastrostomy is inserted into the …….
   a. Stomach
   b. Small intestine
   c. Nose
   d. Small bowel
4. Naso-enteral tubes can be used for ………..
   a. About 4 months
   b. About 9 months
   c. About 12 months
   d. 24 months
5. Which of the following is true about formulas?
   a. It is given at room temperature
   b. It is ordered by the nurse
   c. Opened formula can remain at room temperature for about 16 hours
   d. All of the above
6. Which if the following is true about scheduled feeding?
   a. At least 2 feedings are given each day
   b. Usually 8 to 12 ounces are given over about 2 hours
   c. It is also known as intermittent feeding
   d. A feeding pump is used
7. Which of the following is true about continuous feeding?
   a. It is used specially when there is emergency
   b. A feeding bag is used by the nurse
   c. Feeding is given over 24 hours
   d. At least 4 bags are given each day
8. Which of the following is a risk of tube feeding?
   a. Nausea
   b. Vomiting
   c. Fever
   d. All of the above

9. In continuous feeding the RN checks the tube placement every ....
   a. 1 hour
   b. 4 hours
   c. 8 hours
   d. 12 hours
10. Which of the following is a cause of regurgitation?
   a. Sneezing
   b. Vomiting
   c. Over feeding
   d. All of the above
11. Which of the following should be done when to prevent aspiration during tube feeding?
   a. Position the person in a sims position
   b. Lay the patient on the left side to ease digestion
   c. Let the patient stand for few minutes after feeding
   d. None of the above
12. Which of the following can be done to prevent discomfort for persons using tube feeding?
   a. Give oral hygiene every 30 minutes if the person is awake
   b. Use lubricant for the lips every 2 hours
   c. Perform mouth rinse every 5 hours
   d. All of the above
13. Which of the following should be done when caring for persons using tube feeding?
   a. Do not insert feeding tubes
   b. Syringe or feeding bags should be placed at 50 inches above the stomach
   c. Ensure feeding through syringe in done in about 10 minutes
   d. Use about 150ml of flushing solution for an adult
14. Which of the following is true about parenteral nutrition
   a. It enters the GI tract through the capillaries
   b. Nutrients is giving through a catheter
   c. Food is passed into the small intestine
   d. All of the above
15. Total parenteral nutrition is used when which of the following occurs?
   a. Fever
   b. Difficult breathing
   c. Severe trauma
   d. Diarrhea
16. Doctor order IV therapy to ....
   a. Provide sugar for energy
   b. Give drugs and blood
   c. Replace minerals

d. All of the above

17. Which of the following is a peripheral IV site?
    a. Basilic vein
    b. Subclavian vien
    c. Internal jugular vein
    d. All of the above

18. Which of the following is a central venous site?
    a. Radial vein
    b. Internal jugular vein
    c. Basilic vein
    d. Cephalic vein

19. Which of the following should be done when you hear an alarm from the IV pump?
    a. Adjust the controls on the IV pumps
    b. Change the position of the clamp
    c. Call the nurse
    d. All of the above

20. Which of the following can be done when assisting to care for a person on IV therapy?
    a. Do not move the needle or catheter
    b. Protect the IV bag when the person is walking
    c. Assist the person with turning and re-positioning
    d. All of the above

Section 26

Measuring vital signs

1. Which of the following is a vital sign of body function?
   a. Pulse
   b. Temperature
   c. Blood pressure
   d. All of the above

2. Which of the following affects vital signs?
   a. Anxiety
   b. Sleep
   c. Weather
   d. All of the above

3. ....is the amount of heat in the body
   a. Respirations
   b. Blood pressure
   c. Temperature

d. Pulse

4. Oral temperature are taken when the person ....
   a. Has heart disease
   b. Is under 5 years
   c. Is unconscious
   d. Is paralyzed in one side of the body

5. Which of the following is true about rectal sites?
   a. It should not be used for infants
   b. It should be avoided when a patient is taking oxygen
   c. It should be used when a person has mouth sore
   d. All of the above

6. Which of the following temperature site is non-invasive
   a. Rectal site
   b. Oral site
   c. Temporal artery site
   d. Tympanic membrane site

7. Which of the following is true about glass thermometer?
   a. It is battery operated
   b. It is filled with a substance
   c. It can be used in the ears
   d. All of the above

8. Which of the following is true about disposable oral thermometer?
   a. Chemical dots change color when heated
   b. It is used once
   c. It measures in 45 to 60 seconds
   d. All of the above

9. Which of the following is true about standard electronic thermometers?
   a. A disposable cover protects the probes
   b. The oral red is used for auxiliary temperatures
   c. It measures temperature in 2 to 3 minutes
   d. All of the above

10. ....is used for persons who are confused and resist care
    a. Tympanic membrane thermometers
    b. Glass thermometers
    c. Pacifier thermometer
    d. Disposable oral thermometer

11. The ....pulse is used most often
    a. Temporal
    b. Carotid
    c. Radial
    d. Apical

12. The .... pulse is taken during cardiopulmonary resuscitation

a. Femoral

b. Carotid

c. Apical

d. Radial

13. All of the following is true about stethoscope EXCEPT?

a. It is used to take radial pulse

b. It is used for blood pressures

c. It is used to listen to the sounds from the lungs

d. It makes sound louder

14. The .... Pulse is used for infants and children under 2 years

a. Femoral pulse

b. Apical pulse

c. Carotid pulse

d. Brachial pulse

15. The adult pulse rate is between ....per minute

a. 20 TO 40

b. 30 TO 60

c. 60 TO 100

d. 100 TO 150

16. Apical pulses are taken on persons who .....

a. Have heart disease

b. Have irregular heart rhythms

c. Take drugs that affect the heart

d. All of the above

17. The healthy adults has .... respirations per minute

a. 1 TO 10

b. 5 TO 20

c. 12 TO 20

d. 20 TO 30

18. Which of the following should be done when taking respirations?

a. Inform the person you are taking respirations

b. Count when the person when the person is at rest

c. Count respirations for 2 minutes if you notice abnormalities

d. All of the above

19. Which of the following is an indication of hypertension?

a. When systolic pressure is 100 mm Hg

b. When diastolic pressure is 50 mm Hg

c. When systolic pressure is 140 mm Hg

d. When diastolic pressure is 70 mm Hg

20. Which of the following factors affect blood pressure?

a. Gender

b. Weight

c. Race

d. All of the above

Section 27

Exercise and activity

1. Which of the following causes decreased activity?
   a. Arthritis
   b. Nervous system disorder
   c. Muscular disorder
   d. All of the above
2. ....is the loss of muscle strength from inactivity
   a. Deconditioning
   b. Contracture
   c. Atrophy
   d. Syncope
3. In strict bedrest which if the following is the patient allowed to do?
   a. Self feeding
   b. Bathing
   c. Use commode for elimination
   d. No activity is allowed
4. Which of the following complication can occur from bed rest?
   a. Pressure ulcer
   b. Anemia
   c. Alopecia
   d. Diarrhea
5. A …….. is the lack of joint mobility caused by abnormal shortening of a muscle
   a. Atrophy
   b. Orthostatic hypotension
   c. Contracture
   d. Syncope
6. ....is a brief loss of consciousness
   a. Coma
   b. Syncope

c. Death

d. Postural hypotension

7. Which of the following is true about bed boards?

    a. They are placed on the mattress

    b. They are made of plywood

    c. They prevent plantar flexion

    d. They prevent external rotation

8. Which of the following is used to prevent hips and legs from turning outwards?

    a. Trochanter rolls

    b. Hip abduction wedges

    c. Hand rolls

    d. Splints

9. ....keeps the weight of the top linens off the feet and toes

    a. Bed cradles

    b. Splints

    c. Hip abduction wedges

    d. Footdrop

10. ....is used to keep the hips apart

    a. Trachanter rolls

    b. Bed cradles

    c. Hip abduction wedges

    d. Splints

11. ....is moving a body part away from the mid-line of the body

    a. Abduction

    b. Adduction

    c. Flexion

    d. Extension

12. In .... exercise you move the joints through their range of motion

    a. Active range of motion

    b. Passive range of motion

    c. Active assistive range of motion

    d. All of the above

13. Which of the following is true about crutches?

    a. It is used for weakness on one side of the body

    b. It helps to correct deformity

    c. It is used when persons cannot use one leg

    d. All of the above

14. Which of the following precautions should be followed when a person is using crutches?

    a. Ensure the tips are dry

    b. Tighten all bolts

c. Have the person wear street shoes

d. All of the above

15. Which of the following is true about walkers?

    a. It gives less support than cane

    b. They prevent joint movement

    c. They have wheels on the front legs

    d. It corrects deformities

Section 28

Comfort, Rest and Sleep

1. Which of the following is an OBRA requirement of how a room should be?

    a. No more than 5 people in a room

    b. An odor free room

    c. A room temperature between 81⬚F and 95⬚F

    d. All of the above

2. ………is felt suddenly from injury, disease or trauma

    a. Acute pain

    b. Chronic pain

    c. Mild pain

    d. Phantom pain

3. ………. Continues for a long time or occurs on and off

    a. Radiating pain

    b. Continuous pain

    c. Chronic pain

    d. Phantom pain

4. Which of the following is true about radiating pain?

    a. Arthritis is a common cause

    b. It lessens with healing

    c. It is felt at the site of tissue damage and in nearby areas

    d. It lasts for a short time

5. ………is felt in body parts that is no longer there

    a. Phantom pain

    b. Chronic pain

    c. Radiating pain

    d. Acute pain

6. Which of the following factors affects pain?

    a. Anxiety

b. Culture

c. Past experience

d. All of the above

7. Which of the following helps to reduce pain?

   a. Lack of rest

   b. Anxiety

   c. Busy activities

   d. All of the above

8. Which of the following is a sign or symptom of pain?

   a. Weakness

   b. Crying

   c. Pacing

   d. All of the above

9. Which of the following promotes rest?

   a. Noisy environment

   b. Bright lights

   c. Good alignment

   d. Cluttered room

10. ....is a state of unconsciousness, reduced voluntary muscle activity and lowered metabolism a. Sleep

   b. Death

   c. Rest

   d. Relaxation

11. Which of the following is true about sleep?

   a. It lets the body and mind rest

   b. It refreshes and renews the person

   c. Vital signs are lower when awake

   d. All of the above

12. Which of the following is true about the Non REM sleep?

   a. The person is hard to arouse

   b. It has four stages

   c. Mental restoration occurs

   d. Events of the day are reviewed

13. Which of the following is true about stage one of Non REM sleep?

   a. Lasts 10 to 20 minutes

   b. It is the lightest sleep

   c. The person rarely moves

   d. Sleep working may occur

14. Which of the following is the deepest stage of sleep

   a. Stage 2

   b. Stage 3

   c. Stage 4

d. Stage 5

15. ....is a chronic condition in which the person cannot sleep or stay asleep all night
    a. Sleep deprivation
    b. Sleepwalking
    c. Insomnia
    d. Fatigue

Section 29

Admission, Transfers and Discharges

1. ....is the official departure of a person from a health care setting
    a. Transfer
    b. Discharge
    c. Admission
    d. Removal

2. According to the OBRA, which of the following is a reason for transfer or discharge?
    a. The person is tired of the center
    b. The center is closing
    c. The person family members are tired of the center
    d. The center is on fire

3. The admission process usually starts in the ....
    a. Nursing station
    b. Admitting office
    c. Emergency room
    d. Doctor's office

4. Which of the following information is recorded at admission?
    a. Full name
    b. Doctor's name
    c. Religion
    d. All of the above

5. Which of the following should be done upon admission of a new resident?
    a. Give names of the nurses and nursing assistants
    b. Place signal light within reach
    c. Introduce other residents or room mates
    d. All of the above

6. Which of the following procedures should be carried out when preparing a room for a new resident?
    a. If a person arrives by stretcher leave the bed closed
    b. Attach signal light to the bed
    c. Make a surgical bed if the person arrives by wheelchair
    d. All of the above

7. Which of the following should be noted when measuring weight and height?
    a. The person only wears a gown
    b. Slippers can be worn
    c. A wet incontinence product may be worn
    d. After breakfast is the best time to weigh

8. Which of the following should be done before discharging the resident?
    a. The person is taught about diet, exercise and drugs
    b. If leaving by ambulance a wheelchair is used
    c. The nurse must order the person to leave before he is being discharged
    d. All of the above

9. Which of the following should be done after a discharge?
    a. Report the time of discharge
    b. Strip the bed and clean the unit
    c. Make a closed bed
    d. All of the above

10. Which of the following decides who can visit?
    a. The nurse
    b. The patient
    c. The doctor
    d. The family members

Section 30

Assisting with physical examination

1. Physical examinations are done to ....
    a. Promote health
    b. Determine fitness for work
    c. Diagnose disease
    d. All of the above

2. ....is used to examine the mouth, teeth, and throat
    a. Tuning fork
    b. Laryngeal mirror
    c. Mouth stethoscope
    d. Cavity microscope

3. ....is used to examine the inside of the nose
    a. Otoscope
    b. Percussion hammer
    c. Nasal speculum
    d. Turinig fork
4. ....is used to tap body parts to test reflexes
    a. Opthalmoscope
    b. Otoscope
    c. Percussion hammer
    d. Nasal speculum
5. Vaginal speculum is used to ....
    a. Open the vaginal
    b. Expand the vaginal walls
    c. Insert solutions into the vaginal
    d. All of the above
6. ....is vibrated to test hearing
    a. Otoscope
    b. Turning fork
    c. Percussion hammer
    d. Sphygmomanometer
7. Which of the following should be done when preparing a person for examination?
    a. Have the person void to empty bladder
    b. Obtain urine specimen
    c. Measure weight and vital signs
    d. All of the above
8. In the .... the person is supine with legs together
    a. Dorsal recumbent position
    b. Lithotomy position
    c. Knee chest position
    d. Genupectoral position
9. The dorsal recumbent position is used to examine ....
    a. The thighs
    b. The abdomen
    c. The vagina
    d. The rectum
10. The lithotomy position is used to examine the ....
    a. Chest
    b. Knees
    c. Vaginal
    d. Abdomen
11. In ....position the body is flexed about 90 degrees from the hips

a. Genupectoral

b. Sims

c. Lithotomy position

d. Dorsal recumbent position

12. Which of the following is true about the sims position?

a. The person lies on her back

b. The hips are at the edge of the exam table

c. It is used to examine the vagina

d. The person kneels and rests the body on the knee

13. Which of the following should be done when assisting with physical examinations?

a. Provide for privacy

b. Position the person as directed

c. Protect the person from falling

d. All of the above

14. After the examination……….

a. Discard disposable items

b. Label specimens

c. Replace supplies so the tray is ready for the next exam

d. All of the above

15. Which of the following should be done to ease a person's fears before the examination?

a. Show the person the instruments that will be used

b. Position the person immediately

c. Tell the person good things about the examiner

d. Remove the person's clothes

Section 31

Collecting and testing specimens

1. Specimens are collected to ……..disease

a. Treat

b. Detect

c. Prevent

d. All of the above

2. Which of the following should be done when collecting specimens?

a. Label the container at the nursing station

b. Ask the person to void after collecting stool specimen

c. Urine must not contain tissue

d. Place the specimen container in a plastic bag

3. Which of the following is true about random urine specimen?

a. It is collected at a specific time

b. It should be collected mid stream

c. No special measures are needed when collecting

d. All of the above

4. Which of the following is true about the midstream specimen?

a. The perineal are is cleaned before collecting the specimen

b. The urine is chilled on ice

c. It is used for a routine urinalysis

d. No special measures are needed

5. Which of the following should be done to prevent growth of microbes in the specimen?

a. Add ice into the urine

b. Refrigerate the urine

c. Add preservative to the urine

d. Keep the urine in cold water

6. Which of the following is true about 24 hour urine specimen?

a. The person voids to begin the test with an empty bladder

b. Save the first urine measured at the start of the 24 hour collection period

c. The test is restarted if urine is cloudy

d. The test is restarted if urine contains blood

7. ....is used for infants or children who are not toilet trained

a. Catheters

b. Collection bag

c. Urine tube

d. Syringe

8. Usually a child should void after .... of drinking fluids?

a. 5 minute

b. 8 minutes

c. 30 minutes

d. 6 hours

9. Which of the following causes change in the pH level of urine?

a. Illness

b. Food

c. Drugs

d. All of the above

10. In a diabetic patient, ... Is tested in the urine

a. Ketones

b. Acidity

c. Alkaline

d. Blood

11. Test for ketones are usually done …….times a day

    a. 2
    b. 4
    c. 6
    d. 8

12. Calculus can be developed in the …..

    a. Bladder
    b. Kidney
    c. Ureter
    d. All of the above

13. Stools are studied for ……..

    a. Glucose
    b. Acidity
    c. Worms
    d. Stones

14. Which of the following should be done when collecting stools?

    a. Take sample from the middle of a formed stool
    b. Do not include pus or mucus
    c. Freeze the specimen to preserve it
    d. All of the above

15. Sputum specimens are studies for …….

    a. Blood
    b. Fat
    c. Glucose
    d. Ketones

16. Blood glucose testing is used for persons with…..

    a. Tuberculosis
    b. Diarrhea
    c. Diabetes
    d. Heart attack

17. Which of the following is a good puncture site for blood glucose testing?

    a. Index fingers
    b. Thumbs
    c. Ring finger
    d. All of the above

18. Which of the following should be done when carrying out glucose testing?

    a. Discard the glucometer after testing
    b. Do not use discolored strips
    c. The ring finger should be used for infants
    d. All of the above

19. Which of the following should be done when collecting specimen?

a. Allow visitors in the room

b. Close doors for privacy

c. Place specimen in a transparent container

d. All of the above

20. Which of the following should be done after measuring blood glucose?

a. Discard used supplies

b. Complete a safety check of the room

c. Report and record test result

d. All of the above

Section 32

The person having surgery

1. Surgery can be done to ......

a. Replace a tumor

b. Relieve symptoms

c. Improve appearance

d. All of the above

2. .... is done by choice to improve the person's well being

a. Emergency surgery

b. Urgent surgery

c. Elective surgery

d. Compulsory surgery

3. ....is done to save a life or function

a. Urgent surgery

b. Elective surgery

c. Emergency surgery

d. Scheduled surgery

4. Which of the following is an example of elective surgery?

a. Joint replacement surgery

b. Cancer surgery

c. Coronary artery bypass surgery

d. All of the above

5. Which of the following is a common fear of surgical patients?

a. Disability

b. Cancer

c. Pain

d. All of the above

6. ....is where the person wakes up after surgery

a. Post anesthesia care unit

b. Emergency unit

c. Surgical unit

d. Recovery unit

7. Which of the following is done immediately after surgery?

a. Ambulation

b. Leg exercise

c. Fluid administration

d. Voiding

8. Repositioning and turning should be done at least every…..after surgery

a. 1 hour

b. 4 hours

c. 6 hours

d. 12 hours

9. Which of the following test is often ordered before surgery?

b. Blood glucose

c. Stool testing

d. Urinalysis

e. Hormonal testing

10. The person is not allowed to feed through the mouth …….before surgery

a. 24 hours

b. 16 hours

c. 8 hours

d. 2 hours

11. Which of the following is ordered before bowel surgery?

a. Chest x-rays

b. Enemas

c. Urinalysis

d. Blood glucose

12. Which of the following is allowed in the surgery room?

a. Fake nails

b. Operating gown

c. Hair clips

d. Jewelry

13. Which of the following surgeries can cause swelling of the fingers?

a. Breast surgeries

b. Arm surgeries

c. Shoulder surgeries

d. All of the above

14. Which of the following is done to prep the skin before the surgery?

a. Remove hair at and around the site

b. Remove eyeglasses

c. Remove contact lenses

d. Remove dentures

15. Which of the following is needed before surgery is done?

    a. The person's consent

    b. The doctor's consent

    c. The family's consent

    d. The facility's consent

16. ....is responsible for securing written consent

    a. The nurse

    b. The doctor

    c. The nursing assistant

    d. The family members

17. Pre-operative drugs are given to ....

    a. Help the person stay alive

    b. Keep the person awake

    c. Prevent vomiting

    d. Reduce surgery time

18. ......is a loss of feeling or sensation produced by a drug

    a. Anesthesia

    b. Sedation

    c. Sleep

    d. Calmness

19. ....is a loss of feeling or sensation in a small area

    a. General anesthesia

    b. Local anesthesia

    c. Regional anesthesia

    d. Internal anesthesia

20. All of the following is done to prepare the person's room after surgery EXCEPT

    a. Lower the bed rails

    b. Move furniture's out of the way

    c. Make a closed bed

    d. Place equipments and supplies in the room

21. Measure vital signs and pulse oximetry and observe the person every ....until the person's condition is stable a. 15 minutes

    b. 60 minutes

    c. 2 hours

    d. 4 hours

22. Which of the following should be observed?

    a. Confusion

    b. Nausea

    c. Pain

d. All of the above

23. ....helps prevent respiratory complication
    a. Coughing
    b. Leg exercise
    c. Repositioning
    d. Sleeping

24. An.............is a blod clot that travels through the vascular system until it lodges in the blood vessels a. Thrombus
    b. Embolus
    c. Villi
    d. Atelectasis

25. Which of the following prevents thrombi?
    a. Deep breathing
    b. Coughing
    c. Leg exercise
    d. Sleeping

26. Which of the following is true about leg exercises?
    a. They increase venous blood flow
    b. They are prevent blood clot
    c. They are done at least every 1 hour to 2 hours
    d. All of the above

27. Which of the following should be noted when applying bandages?
    a. Let the bandage be loose
    b. Start work in the top part and work towards the distal part
    c. Expose fingers or toes
    d. All of the above

28. A ....is a sleeve that wraps around the leg
    a. Bandage
    b. Sequential compression device
    c. Elastic stocks
    d. None of the above

29. Early ambulation prevents which of the following complications?
    a. Pneumonia
    b. Infection
    c. Evisceration
    d. Hemorrhage

30. The person must void within .... after surgery
    a. 1
    b. 2
    c. 4
    d. 8

Section 33

Wound care

1. ......is a partial thickness wound caused by the scraping away or rubbing of the skin
   a. Incision
   b. Abrasion
   c. Ulcer
   d. Excoriation

2. An ....is a cut produced surgically a sharp instrument used to creates an opening into an organ a. Puncture wound
   b. Contusion
   c. Incision
   d. Abrasion

3. In ....the tissues are injured but the skin is not broken
   a. Open wound
   b. Closed wound
   c. Unintentional wound
   d. Intentional wound

4. ....is a shallow or deep crater like sore of the skin or a mucous membrane a. Ulcer
   b. Puncture wound
   c. Incision
   d. Contusion

5. Which of the is an example of closed wound ?
   a. Bruises
   b. Twists
   c. Sprains
   d. All of the above

6. Which of the following is true about clean wound?
   a. It is not infected
   b. It has a risk of infection
   c. Tissues may show sign of inflammation
   d. All of the above

7. ....wound contains large amount of microbe and shows sign of infection
   a. Chronic wound
   b. Clean wound
   c. Infected wound
   d. Open wound

8. In ....the dermis, epidermis, and subcutaneous tissue are penetrated
   a. Full thickness wound

b. Extreme thickness wound

c. Partial thickness wound

d. Reduced thickness wound

9. Which of the following is true about skin tears?

    b. It is made from surgical sharp instrument

    c. It is created from therapy

    d. The epidermis separates from the underlying tissues

    e. It affects the subcutaneous tissues

10. Which of the following causes skin tear

    a. Friction

    b. Shearing

    c. Pulling

    d. All of the above

11. Which of the following can be done to prevent skin tears?

    a. Dress and undress the person carefully

    b. Keep your fingernails short and smoothly filed

    c. Do not wear bracelets

    d. All of the above

12. ......is swelling caused by fluid collecting in tissues

    a. Gangrene

    b. Edema

    c. Thrombosis

    d. Laceration

13. Which of the following measures can be used to prevent circulatory ulcers?

    a. Rub the skin during bathing

    b. Dress the person carefully

    c. Do not dress the person in tight clothes

    d. Do not apply adhesive tape

14. ....are open sores on the lower legs on the feet caused poor venous blood flow

    a. Diabetic foot ulcer

    b. Venous ulcer s

    c. Gangrene

    d. Arterial ulcers

15. Which of the following is true about venous ulcer?

    a. Infection is a risk

    b. It is caused by poor arterial blood flow

    c. Healing is fast

    d. All of the above

16. Which of the following is a risk factor for venous ulcer?

    a. Advanced age

    b. Obesity

   c. Decreased mobility

   d. All of the above

17. ....is a risk factor for arterial ulcer

   a. Altered mental awareness

   b. Poor hydration

   c. Smoking

   d. Old age

18. Which of the following is true about diabetic foot ulcer?

   a. Gangrene is a risk

   b. Blood flow increase

   c. Sore heals rapidly

   d. All of the above

19. ......are thick layers of skin caused by too much rubbing or pressure on the same spot.

   a. Blisters

   b. Corns and calluses

   c. Bunions

   d. Hammer toes

20. ....is a big toe slanting towards the small toes

   a. Hammer toes

   b. Plantar warts

   c. Bunions

   d. Ingrown toenails

21. Which of the following is true about plantar warts?

   a. They occur on soles

   b. They occur in between the toe nails

   c. It is caused by bacteria

   d. It heals rapidly

22. ....is a fungus causing redness and cracked skin between the toes and on the bottom of the feet a. Athlete foot

   b. Blisters

   c. Cracked skin

   d. Hammer toes

23. Which of the following is true about dry and cracked skin?

   a. The foot does not receive message from the brain

   b. It is caused by virus

   c. Toenails become yellow

   d. All of the above

24. Which of the following occurs in the first phase of wound healing?

   a. The scar gains strength

   b. Proliferation occurs in the cell

   c. Bleeding stops

d. Red scar becomes pale

25. Which of the following is true about first intention type of wound healing?
    a. It is for contaminated and infected wounds
    b. The wound is closed
    c. It usually leaves a large scar
    d. Healing takes longer

26. Which of the following prolongs healing?
    a. Smoking
    b. Diabetes
    c. Circulatory disease
    d. All of the above

27. Which of the following is a complication that may result from wounds?
    a. Infection
    b. Hemorrhage
    c. Shock
    d. All of the above

28. Which of the following is true about serous drainage?
    a. It is a clear watery fluid
    b. It contains blood or traces of blood
    c. It is thick and brownish
    d. It contains blood cell platelets

29. Which of the following is true about drainage?
    a. It must leave the wound for healing
    b. Trapped drainage causes swelling
    c. It drainage does not flow out complications can occur
    d. All of the above

30. Which of the following is a function of wound dressing?
    a. To beautify the wound
    b. It reduces pain in the wound area
    c. It helps absorb drainage
    d. It is reduces the smell of the wound

Pressure ulcers

1. ....is an area where the bone sticks out or projects from the flat surface of the body
    a. Bony prominence
    b. Shear
    c. Friction

d. Eschar

2. ………is when the skin remains in place and the underlying tissues move and stretch and tear underlying capillaries a. Friction
   b. Shear
   c. Bony prominence
   d. Pressure ulcer

3. Which of the following is true about unavoidable pressure ulcer?
   a.   It develops from the improper use of the nursing process
   b.   It occurs despite efforts to prevent it from occurring
   c.   It is mostly brought from home
   d.   It occurs when the center does not identify the person as a risk 4. Which of the following are causes of skin breakdown?
   a. Poor nutrition
   b. Poor hydration
   c. Dryness
   d. All of the above

5. Which of the following is a risk factor of pressure ulcers in children?
   a. Circulatory problems
   b. Inability to sense pain
   c. Epidermal stripping
   d. Lowered mental awareness

6. Which of the following is true about stage one of pressure ulcer?
   a. The skin is intact with redness over bony prominence
   b. There is partial thickness skin loss
   c. Slough may be present
   d. Eschar may be present

7. Which of the following is true about stage 4 of pressure ulcer?
   a. The skin becomes very red
   b. Blister may be open
   c. Eschar may appear
   d. The ulcer is reddish or pink

8. The skin is intact in stage ……
   a. One
   b. Two
   c. Three
   d. Four

9. Pressure occurs mostly on the ……..
   a. Shoulder
   b. Heel
   c. Arm
   d. Fingers

10. Which of the following can prevent pressure ulcers?
    a. Position the person on tubes or medical devices
    b. Reposition chairfast persons every 4 hours
    c. Powder sheets lightly
    d. Massage over pressure point
11. Which of the following is true about bed cradle?
    a. It is made of foam
    b. It is a metal frame placed on the bed and over the person
    c. It distributes the persons weight evenly over the bed
    d. All of the above
12. ....raises the heel and foot off the bed
    a. Heel and foot elevator
    b. Heel and foot protector
    c. Gel pads
    d. Bed cradle
13. Which of the following is true about eggcrate type pads?
    a. Air flows within it
    b. It is useful for persons with spinal cord injury
    c. Peaks in the pad distribute the person's weight more evenly
    d. All of the above
14. ....decides what dressing to use
    a. Nurse
    b. Doctor
    c. Patient
    d. Nursing assistant
15. Which of the following is true pressure ulcers
    a. The dressing applied on it must be very moist
    b. It is colonized with bacteria from stages 2 to 4
    c. Pain and delayed healing does not signal infection
    d. All of the above

Section 35

Heat and cold applications

1. Which of the following is a function of heat?
    a. It relieves pain
    b. It relaxes muscles

c. It promotes healing

d. All of the above

2. Which of the following occurs when heat is applied to the skin?

    a. The skin becomes numb

    b. It constricts the blood vessels

    c. Tissues have more oxygen

    d. All of the above

3. Hot applications are usually used to treat ......

    a. Arthritis

    b. Gangrene

    c. Fever

    d. Burns

4. Which of the following should be noted when applying heat?

    a. It can result in burns

    b. Prolonged heat application can cause blood flow to decrease

    c. Metal implants pose a risk when applying heat

    d. All of the above

5. In sitz bath, which of the following is immersed into water?

    a. The rectal area

    b. The foot

    c. The lower arm

    d. The lower leg

6. Which of the following is true about heat application?

    a. The dry heat penetrates more deeply than moist heat

    b. Dry heat needs higher temperature

    c. Dry heat has greater effect

    d. All of the above

7. Which of the following is an example of dry heat application?

    a. Hot compress

    b. Hot soak

    c. Aquathermia pad

    d. Sitz bath

8. Which of the following is true about cold application?

    a. It increases blood flow

    b. It makes blood vessels dilate

    c. They are useful immediately after an injury

    d. It increases fever

9. Which of the following should be done when applying hot or cold pads?

    a. Do not apply very hot application

    b. Provide for privacy

    c. Do not let the person change the temperature

    d. All of the above

10. Which of the following is true about hypothermia?
   a. It is often caused by hot weather
   b. The person is warmed to prevent death
   c. Body temperature is greater than 103□F
d.   It can be caused by dehydration

Section 36

Oxygen needs

1. Which of the following is true about oxygen?
   a. It is a gas
   b. It is a basic need required for life
   c. It has no color
   d. All of the above
2. Air enters the body through the ....
   a. Nose
   b. Pharynx
   c. Larynx
   d. Trachea
3. ....picks up oxygen from thee alveoli
   a. Lungs
   b. Blood in the capillaries
   c. Bronchioles
   d. Pleura
4. Which of the following causes oxygen needs to increase?
   a. Exercise
   b. Fever
   c. Pain
   d. All of the above
5. ....is when breathing stops
   a. Respiratory arrest
   b. Respiratory depression
   c. Respiratory stop
   d. Respiratory concentration
6. Which of the following affects respiratory rate?
   a. Brain damage
   b. Narcotics
   c. Red blood cell count

d. All of the above

7. Which of the following produce red blood cell?
   a. Vitamin C
   b. Vitamin D
   c. Vitamin K
   d. Vitamin E

8. ....is known as tachypnea
   a. No breathing
   b. Slow breathing
   c. Rapid breathing
   d. Deep respiration

9. ....means that the cells do not have enough oxygen
   a. Dyspnea
   b. Hypoxia
   c. Bradypnea
   d. Hypoventilation

10. ....is an early sign of hypoxia
    a. Restlessness
    b. Dyspnea
    c. Apnea
    d. Constipation

11. ....breathing is slow, shallow and sometimes irregular
    a. Cheyne stokes respiration
    b. Kussmaul respiration
    c. Hypoventilation
    d. Hyperventilation

12. Which of the following is true about bradypnea?
    a. It occur suddenly
    b. Respirations are fewer than 12 per minutes
    c. Pregnancy is a cause
    d. All of the above

13. Which of the following is a sign of hypoxia?
    a. Agitation
    b. Fatigue
    c. Anxiety
    d. All of the above

14. Which of the following is true about orthopnea?
    a. The person breathes comfortably only while sitting
    b. Breathing is painful
    c. Breathing is slow
    d. All of the above

15. ....are rapid and deep respirations followed 10 to 30 seconds of apnea

a. Kussmaul respirations

b. Biot's respirations

c. Cheyne stokes respiration

d. None of the above

16. Which of the following is a common cause of orthopnea?

a. Pneumonia

b. Asthma

c. Emphysema

d. All of the above

17. Which of the following is used to check the airway structure for bleeding and tumor?

a. Chest x-ray

b. Lung scan

c. Bronchoscopy

d. Thoracentesis

18. ....measures the amount of air moving into and out of the lungs

a. Chest x-rays

b. Bronchoscopy

c. Thoracentesis

d. Pulmonary function test

19. Which of the following is a sign and symptoms of altered respiratory function

a. Cyanosis

b. Chest pain

c. Shortness of breath

d. All of the above

20. The normal range of oxygen concentration in the blood is around ....

a. 60% to 70%

b. 70% to 80%

c. 85% to 95%

d. 95% to 100%

21. ....is used to measure the oxygen concentration in the arterial blood

a. Pulse oximetry

b. Bronchoscopy

c. Thoracentesis

d. Lung scan

22. Breathing is easier in ....position

a. Lateral

b. Semi fowler

c. Prone

d. Sims

23. Which of the following promotes oxygenation?

a. Deep breathing
b. Coughing exercise
c. Aerobic exercise
d. All of the above

24. Which of the following is true about oxygen tank?
    a. It removes oxygen from the air
    b. It is filled from a statutory unit
    c. It is placed by the bedside
    d. It allows the person to be mobile

25. Which of the following is true about venturi mask?
    a. Precise amounts of oxygen are given
    b. The prongs are inserted into the nostrils
    c. A band goes behind the ears and nose
d.   All of the above

Section 37

Respiratory support and therapies

1. ....is inserted through the mouth and into the pharynx
    a. Oropharyngeal airway
    b. Endotracheal tube
    c. Trancheostomy tube
    d. Osotomy tube

2. ......is inserted through the mouth or nose and into the trachea
    a. Tracheostomy tube
    b. Endotracheal tube
    c. Osotomy tube
    d. Oropharyngeal airway

3. ......performs tracheostomies
    a. Registered Nurse
    b. Doctors
    c. LPN
    d. LVN

4. Which of the following may require permanent tracheostomy?
    a. Brain damage
    b. Cancer
    c. Severe airway trauma
    d. All of the above

5. Which of the following is true about obturator?
   a. It keeps the airway patent
   b. It keeps the tracheostomy
   c. It has a round end
   d. It is secured with a velcro
6. Which of the following is true about the outer cannula?
   a. It is removed for cleaning
   b. It is taped to the wall
   c. It keeps the tracheostomy patent
   d. All of the above
7. Which of the following safety measure should be adhered to when using tracheostmies?
   a. The stoma is covered when outdoors
   b. The preferred form of bath is by shower
   c. Swimming is allowed once in a while
   d. All of the above
8. Which of the following could occur from retained secretions?
   a. It can obstruct air flow into and out of the airway
   b. It provides an environment for microbes
   c. It interferes with oxygen and carbon dioxide exchange
   d. All of the above
9. To suction the lower airway, the suction catheter is passed through the........
   a. Nose
   b. Tracheostomy tube
   c. Mouth
   d. Pharynx
10. Which of the following is true about sunctions?
    a. The yankauer suction catheter is often used for small and tiny secretions
    b. The lungs are hyperventilated before suctioning through the mouth
    c. A suction source is needed
    d. The ambu bag is attached to the mouth
11. Which of the following complication can occur from suctioning?
    a. Cardiac arrest
    b. Hypoxia
    c. Infection
    d. All of the above
12. Which of the following safety measures should be noted when assisting with suctioning?
    a. The nurse waits 20 to 30 seconds between each suction
    b. Suction is applied while inserting the catheter into the lower airway
    c. For infants the suction cycle is no more than 15 seconds
    d. For adults a suction cycle should not take more than 60 seconds

13. ....is using a machine to move air into and out of the lungs
    a. Mechanical ventilation
    b. Systematic ventilation
    c. Chest tubes insertion
    d. None of the above
14. ....is air in the pleural space
    a. Hemothorax
    b. Pneumothorax
    c. Pleural effusion
    d. Pleural excretion
15. Which of the following is done when giving care to a person with chest tubes?
    a. Prevent tubing kinks
    b. Turn and position the person as directed
    c. Keep the drainage system below the chest

Section 38

Rehabilitation and restorative nursing care

1. Which of the following is true about an acute problem?
    a. The problem cannot be cured
    b. It has a short course
    c. It is controlled
    d. All of the above
2. Which of the following health problems require rehabilitation?
    a. Amputation
    b. Birth defects
    c. Stroke
    d. All of the above
3. Which of the following is true about rehabilitation?
    a. It takes longer in children than any other age group
    b. It cannot be carried out by a nursing assistant
    c. It promotes self-care
    d. The goal is to treat the disorder
4. Rehabilitation starts when the person ......
    a. First seeks health care
    b. First sees the doctor
    c. First starts physical therapy

d. First pays for therapy

5. ………is common for musculo skeletal problems
   a. Physical therapy
   b. Relaxation therapy
   c. Pharmacotherapy
   d. Bladder training

6. …….is the total or partial loss of the ability to use or understand language
   a. Dysphagia
   b. Alopecia
   c. Aphasia
   d. Dyspnea

7. Which of the following is needed for a person with dsyphagia?
   a. Speech therapy
   b. Enteral nutrition
   c. Physical therapy
   d. Pharmacotherapy

8. Which of the following is a social consequence of disability?
   a. Low self esteem
   b. Depression
   c. Anger
   d. All of the above

9. Which of the following can be done to help with rehabilitation or restorative care?
   a. Do not focus on disabilities
   b. Do not give sympathy
   c. Encourage the person to perform
   d. All of the above

10. ………is done for heart disorders
    a. Cardiac rehabilitation
    b. Stroke rehabilitation
    c. Respiratory rehabilitation
    d. Spinal cord rehabilitation

Section 39

Hearing, speech, and vision problems

1. Which of the following is a common cause of vision and hearing loss?
   a. Birth defects
   b. Accidents
   c. Diseases
   d. All of the above

2. The outer part of the ear is called ....
   a. Auricle
   b. Auditory canal
   c. Stapes
   d. Cochlea
3. Glands in the auditory canal secretes a waxy substance called ....
   a. Gel
   b. Cerumen
   c. Serum
   d. Tympanic mucus
4. The inner ear consist of ....
   a. Pinna
   b. Auricle
   c. Cochlea
   d. Lobe
5. Otitis media is infection of the ....ear
   a. Outer
   b. Middle
   c. Inner
   d. Whole
6. Which of the following is true about otitis media?
   a. It is not a chronic disease
   b. Permanent hearing loss can occur
   c. It is not caused by viruses
   d. All of the above
7. ....is a ringing, roaring, hissing, or buzzing sound in the ears or head
   a. Tinnitus
   b. Vertigo
   c. Meniere's disease
   d. Otitis media
8. Which of the following is a signal of otitis media?
   a. Fever
   b. Fluid draining from the ear
   c. Problems sleeping
   d. All of the above
9. Meniere's disease involves the ....ear
   a. Inner
   b. Middle
   c. Outer
   Whole
10. Which of the following is true about meniere's disease?
   a. Symptoms develop overtime

b. Both ears are usually affected

c. An attack can last several hours

d. All of the above

11. ....causes whirling and spinning sensations

   a. Deafness

   b. Vertigo

   c. Pain

   d. Cerumen

12. Which of the following decrease fluid in the inner ear?

   a. Alcohol

   b. Caffeine

   c. Low salt diet

   d. High sodium diet

13. Which of the following should be adhered to when caring for a person with Meniere's disease?

   a. The person should turn his or head at least every 15 minutes

   b. The person must lie down

   c. Bright and glaring lights should be allowed in the room

   d. The person should be allowed to walk independently

14. ....is hearing loss in which it is impossible for the person to understand speech through hearing alone a. Deafness

   b. Tinnitus

   c. Vertigo

   d. Otitis media

15. Which of the following is true about hearing loss?

   a. It occurs in all age group

   b. It is more common in women than men

   c. It occurs more in young people than old people

   d. All of the above

16. Which of the following is a cause of hearing loss?

   a. Head injuries

   b. Stroke

   c. Tumors

   d. All of the above

17. Removing earwax is the duty of the ....

   a. Family members

   b. Patient

   c. Doctor

   d. Nursing assistant

18. Which of the following is a sign of hearing loss?

   a. Speaking too loudly

   b. Leaning forward to hear

c. Asking for words to be repeated

All of the above

19. Which of the following is true about hearing aids?
    a. They make sounds louder
    b. They correct hearing problems
    c. They restore hearing
    d. Hearing ability improves

20. Which of the following measures promote hearing?
    a. Reduce or eliminate background noises
    b. Provide a quiet place to talk
    c. Speak clearly and slowly
    d. All of the above

21. A person with ....of speech cannot use the speech muscles for understanding speech a. Aphasia
    b. Apraxia
    c. Dysarthria
    d. Broca's aphasia

22. Which of the following is true about dysarthria?
    a. The person understands speech and knows what to say
    b. Drooling can occur
    c. The motor speech area in the brain is damaged
    d. All of the above

23. Which of the following is a cause of aphasia?
    a. Cancer
    b. Brain infections
    c. Stroke
    d. All of the above

24. ....relates to difficulty expressing or sending out thoughts
    a. Receptive aphasia
    b. Global aphasia
    c. Expressive aphasia
    d. Mixed aphasia

25. Which of the following is true about receptive aphasia?
    a. The person has problem understanding
    b. Thinking is clear
    c. The person knows what to say
    d. All of the above

26. All of the following should be done when communicating with a speech impaired person EXCEPT
    a. Use short simple sentences
    b. Give full attention
    c. Correct the person's speech

d. Write down key words as needed

27. ……..is the clouding of the lens
    a. Blindness
    b. Cataracts
    c. Glaucoma
       Retinopathy

28. Which of the following is a sign and symptom of cataracts?
    a. Halos around lights
    b. Poor vision at night
    c. Dimmed vision
    d. All of the above

29. Which of the following causes cataracts?
    a. Diabetes
    b. Head injuries
    c. Antibiotics
    d. Brain damage

30. Which of the following is true about glaucoma?
    a. It causes damage to the optic nerve
    b. It is the clouding of the lens
    c. It can be treated through surgery
    d. Prior damage can be reserved through surgery

31. In diabetic retinopathy, the tiny blood vessels in the ……….are damaged
    a. Optic nerve
    b. Retina
    c. Lens
    d. Pupil

32. Which of the following is true about diabetic retinopathy?
    a. Everyone with diabetes is a risk
    b. It usually affects the two eyes
    c. The person needs to control diabetes
    d. All of the above

33. Which of the following is true about age related macular degeneration?
    a. It clouds the lens of the eye
    b. Age is not a risk factor
    c. It blurs central vision
    d. Men are at greater risk

34. Which of the following is a risk factor for age related macular degeneration?
    a. Smoking
    b. Obesity
    c. Family history
    d. All of the above

35. Which of the following is true about low vision?

a. It can be corrected with eyeglasses

b. It can be corrected by surgery

c. Diabetes is a risk factor

d. All of the above

36. Which of the following can be used to help a person with low vision?

    a. Magnifying aids for close vision

    b. Telescopic aids for far vision

    c. Prescription reading glasses

    d. All of the above

37. Which of the following is a sign of vision problems?

    a. Eyes hurting

    b. Vomiting

    c. Constipation

    d. Fever

38. Which of the following should be done when caring for the blind and visually impaired?

    a. Re-arrange furniture and equipment

    b. Tell the person when lights are on are off

    c. Change places where things are kept

    d. Use plates, napkins, placemats, and tablecloths with patterns and design

39. Which of the following is true about Braille?

    a. It read by moving the hands from right to the left along the Braille

    b. The first 10 letters also represent the number 0 to 9

    c. Braille keyboards are not available

    d. All of the above

40. Which of the following should be done when caring for a blind and visually impaired person?

    a. Guide the person in front of you

    b. Grab the person's arm while walking

    c. Provide visual and adaptive device

    d. All of the above

Cancer, immune system, and skin disorders

1. Which of the following is true about benign tumors?
   a. They invade other body parts
   b. They grow to a large size
   c. They are life threatening
   d. All of the above
2. Which of the following is a sign and symptom of brain tumor
   a. Seizures
   b. Pelvic pain
   c. Hematuria
   d. Fatigue
3. Which of the following is a sign and symptom of breast cancer?
   a. A change in breast size
   b. Discharge from the nipple
   c. A lump or thickening in or near the breast
   d. All of the above
4. ....is a sign and symptom of cancer in the kidney
   a. Pelvic pain
   b. Constipation
   c. Weight loss
   d. Dyspnea
5. A cough that gets worse or does not go away is a sign of ....
   a. Fever
   b. Chest pain
   c. Lung cancer
   d. Colon cancer
6. A sore throat or trouble swallowing for more than 6 weeks is a sign of ....
   a. Larynx cancer
   b. Lung cancer
   c. Lymphoma cancer
   d. Brain tumor
7. ....is the most common form of childhood cancer
   a. Brain tumor
   b. Leukemia
   c. Liver cancer
   d. Kidney cancer
8. Which of the following is true about cancer?
   a. Childhood cancer have a high cure rate
   b. Childhood cancer often occur suddenly
   c. It is the second leading cause of death
   d. All of the above

9. Most cancers occur in persons age ....
    a. 1 to 5 years
    b. 6 to 12 years
    c. 15 to 35 years
    d. 65 years above
10. Which of the following is a risk factor for cancer?
    a. Tobacco
    b. Sunlight
    c. Ionizing radiation
    d. All of the above
11. Which of the following is true about surgery as a form of cancer treatment?
    a. It is done to remove tumors
    b. It may result in hair loss
    c. Burns can occur
    d. All of the above
12. ....involves drugs that kill cells
    a. Surgery
    b. Radiation therapy
    c. Chemotherapy
    d. Hormone therapy
13. Which of the following is a side effect of hormone therapy?
    a. Loss of sexual desire
    b. Diarrhea
    c. Stomatitis
    d. Alopecia
14. ....helps the immune system fight the cancer
    a. Chemotherapy
    b. Biological therapy
    c. Hormone therapy
    d. Radiation therapy
15. ....is a example of alternative medicine
    a. Stem cell transplant
    b. Immunotherapy
    c. Acupuncture
    d. All of the above
16. ....is an autoimmune disorder
    a. Lupus
    b. Shingles
    c. Acquired immunodeficiency syndrome
    d. All of the above
17. In ....the immune system attacks the thyroid gland
    a. Lupus

b. Graves disease

c. Multiple sclerosis

d. Rheumatoid arthritis

18. Which of the following is true about lupus?

   a. The thyroid gland produces excess thyroxine

   b. The person has bulging eyeballs

   c. It is an inflammatory disease

   d. All of the above

19. ....are white blood cells that digest and destroy microorganisms and other unwanted substances a. Lymphocytes

   b. Phagocytes

   c. Antigens

   d. Antibodies

20. ....are cells that destroy invading cells

   a. T lymphocytes

   b. B lymphocytes

   c. Phagocytes

   d. Antigens

21. Which of the following is true about autoimmune disorders?

   a. Most of the disorder are chronic

   b. The immune system attacks the body's own normal cells

   c. Fever is a common symptom is all the disorders

   d. All of the above

22. Which of the following is a sign of AIDS

   a. Cough

   b. Fever

   c. Headache

   d. All of the above

23. HIV is spread through ....

   a. Sweat

   b. Breast milk

   c. Saliva

   d. Coughing

24. Which of the following should be done when caring for a person with AIDS

   a. Measure weight daily

   b. Provide oral fluids

   c. Prevent pressure ulcers

   d. All of the above

25. Which of the following is true about shingles?

   a. It is caused by bacteria

   b. It is most common in children

   c. Persons who have had chicken pox are at risk

d.   It can be transferred through sex

Section 41

Nervous system and Musculo-skeletal disorders

1. ....occurs when blood vessel in the brain bursts
   a. Stroke
   b. Parkinson's disease
   c. Multiple sclerosis
   d. Amyotrophic lateral sclerosis
2. Which of the following is true about stroke?
   a. It is the number one cause of death in the united states
   b. It is the leading cause of disability in adults
   c. It occurs in all age group
   d. All of the above
3. Which of the following is a risk factor for strokes?
   a. Diabetes
   b. High blood pressure
   c. Heart disease
   d. All of the above
4. Which of the following is a warning sign of stroke?
   a. Slow movement
   b. Dizziness
   c. Sudden trouble walking
   d. Fatigue
5. Which of the following should be done when caring for a person with stroke?
   a. Turn and re-position the person at least every 2 hours
   b. Encourage incentive spirometry and deep breathing
   c. Do not rush the person
   d. All of the above
6. Which of the following is true about Parkinson's disease?
   a. It occurs in all age groups
   b. It has no cure
   c. It is caused by a blood clot blocks blood flow to the brain
   d. It is the second leading cause of death in the united state 7. Which of the following is a sign of Parkinson's disease?
   a. Slow movements
   b. Severe headache

c. Diarrhea

d. Hemiplegia

8. Which of the following is true about multiple sclerosis?

   a. It is a terminal disease

   b. Symptoms usually start between the ages of 40 to 60

   c. There is no cure

   d. All of the above

9. Which of the following is a sign of multiple sclerosis?

   a. Dizziness

   b. Fatigue

   c. Tremors

   d. All of the above

10. Amyotrophic lateral sclerosis is commonly called ……….

    a. Brain attack

    b. Lou Gehrig's disease

    c. Paralysis

    d. Hemiplegia

11. Which of the following is true about amyotrophic lateral sclerosis?

    a. It is common in women

    b. It is also called cerebro-vascular accident

    c. Most die 3 to 5 years after onset

    d. All of the above

12. Which of the following occurs in amyotrophic lateral sclerosis?

    a. The person cannot move the arms

    b. Muscles for breathing are not affected

    c. The memory decreases

    d. Bowel and bladder functions are altered

13. Which of the following is a cause of traumatic brain injury?

    a. Motor vehicle crashes

    b. Recreational injuries

    c. Sport injuries

    d. All of the above

14. ……..is when the person is unconscious and unaware of surroundings

    a. Stupor

    b. Vegetative state

    c. Persistent vegetative state

    d. Sleep state

15. Persistent vegetative state is when a person is in a vegetative state for more than …….

    a. 1 month

    b. 2 months

    c. 6 months

d. 12 months

16. Which of the following is true about lumbar injuries?
    a. Sensory function in the chest is lost
    b. Muscle function in the arms are lost
    c. The person has paraplegia
    d. All of the above

17. Which of the following is true about thoracic injuries?
    a. Sensory function in the legs are lost
    b. Muscle function in the chest is lost
    c. Muscle function in the trunk is lost
    d. Muscle function in the arm is lost

18. Which of the following occurs when there is autonomic dysreflexia?
    a. It weaken muscles and causes atrophy
    b. The person needs a ventilator to breath
    c. The brain cannot starts voluntary movements
    d. There is uncontrolled stimulation of the sympathetic nervous system

19. Which of the following is a cause of osteoarthritis?
    a. Aging
    b. Joint injury
    c. Being overweight
    d. All of the above

20. Which of the following is true about osteoarthritis?
    a. It is the most common type of arthritis
    b. It can be reversed with pain relief treatment
    c. Bones become fragile
    d. All of the above

Section 42

Cardiovascular, Respiratory and lymphatic disorder

1. Which of the following is a sign of congenital heart defects?
    a. Poor weight gain
    b. Poor feeding
    c. Fast breathing
    d. All of the above

2. Which of the following is a risk factor for cardiovascular disorder?
    a. Stress
    b. Blood pressure
    c. Lack of exercise
    d. All of the above

3. Which of the following is true about cardiovascular disease?
   a. There is greater risk for women than men
   b. It occurs evenly in all age groups
   c. African American are at greater risk
   d. All of the above

4. Pre-hypertension is when the systolic pressure is between ……..
   a. 140 and 160 mm Hg
   b. 120 and 139 mm Hg
   c. 110 and 120 mm Hg
   d. 100 and 105 mm Hg

5. Which of the following is a common cause of hypertension?
   a. Narrowed blood vessels
   b. Motor vehicle accidents
   c. Brain damage
   d. Parkinson's disease

6. Which of the following is true about hypertension?
   a. Symptoms develop over time
   b. It can lead to stroke
   c. Alcohol should be limited
   d. All of the above

7. In …….the coronary arteries become hardened and narrow
   a. Coronary artery disease
   b. Hypertension
   c. Angina
   d. Myocardial infraction

8. The most common cause of heart disease is ……
   a. Gunshot wounds
   b. Sport injuries
   c. Atherosclerosis
   d. Paralysis

9. Which of the following is a major complication of heart disease?
   a. Dyspnea
   b. Angina
   c. Alopecia
   d. Dysreflexia

10. ……is chest pain from reduced blood flow to part of the heart muscle
   a. Myocardial infarction
   b. Dyspnea
   c. Angina
   d. Hypertension

11. Which of the following is true about angina?
   a. It occurs when the heart needs more oxygen

b. Part of the heart muscle dies

c. Blood flow to the heart is blocked

d. All of the above

12. Which of the following causes angina?

a. Heavy meals

b. Over eating

c. Emotional stress

d. All of the above

13. Myocardial infarction is also called ....

a. Heart attack

b. Coronary occlusion

c. Coronary thrombosis

d. All of the above

14. Which of the following is a sign of myocardial infarction?

a. Dyspnea

b. Constipation

c. Fever

d. Cough

15. Which of the following is true about myocardial infarction?

a. It is chest pain from reduced flow part of the heart muscle

b. A blood clot blocks blood flow in an artery with atherosclerosis

c. The coronary arteries become hardened and narrow

d. It cannot be cured

16. ....is an abnormal heart rhythm

a. Dysrhythmia

b. Heart failure

c. Coronary

d. Acute coronary syndrome

17. Which of the following can be used for life threatening dysrhythmia?

a. Defibrillation

b. Ablation

c. Implantable cardioverter defibrillator

d. Nitroglycerin tablet

18. Chronic obstructive pulmonary disease involves which of the following?

a. Emphysema

b. Asthma

c. Pneumonia

d. Influenza

19. Which of the following is true about chronic bronchitis?

a. The alveoli is enlarge

b. Smoking is the major cause

c. Air is trapped inside the lungs

d. All of the above

20. Which of the following is a sign of symptom of sleep apnea?
    a. Loud snoring
    b. Daytime sleepiness
    c. Dry mouth or sore throat after sleeping
    d. All of the above

Section 43

Digestive and endocrine disorders

1. ....is the most common symptom of gastro esophageal reflux disease
    a. Heartburn
    b. Constipation
    c. Diarrhea
    d. Nausea

2. Which of the following is a risk factor of gastro esophageal reflux disease?
    a. Alcohol use
    b. Smoking
    c. Being over-weight
    d. All of the above

3. Which of the following can cause gastric reflux?
    a. Citrus fruits
    b. Chocolate
    c. Caffeine drinks
    d. All of the above

4. Vomiting large amount of blood can lead to ………
    a. Jaundice
    b. Weight loss
    c. Shock
    d. Skin rash

5. Which of the following is true about diverticular disease?
    a. A ruptured pouch is common
    b. Lower fiber diet is a risk factor
    c. Heartburn is a common symptom
    d. Stomach contents flow back from the stomach to the esophagus 6.
    When feces enters the pouches in the colon, they can become …….
    a. Infected
    b. Blocked
    c. Ruptured

d. All of the above

7. Bile is carried from the ....to the gallbladder
    a. Liver
    b. Pancreas
    c. Cystic duct
    d. Hepatic duct

8. Which of the following is true about gallstones?
    a. It is always small like a grain of sand
    b. It is formed when bile hardens into stone like pieces
    c. Gallstones lodge in the common bile duct
    d. Gallstones are melted with nitroglycerin

9. Which of the following persons are at risk of gallstone?
    b. Pregnant women
    c. Persons under the age of 60
    d. A person who smokes
    e. Persons taking alcohol

10. Which of the following is a symptom and sign of gallstone?
    a. Constipation
    b. Jaundice
    c. Hot flashes
    d. Loss of appetite

11. Which of the following is a sign of hepatitis?
    a. Weight loss
    b. Skin rash
    c. Diarrhea
    d. All of the above

12. Which of the following is at risk for hepatitis A
    a. People who live with an infected person
    b. People who received blood products before 1987
    c. People who received blood products before 1992
    d. Hemodialysis patient

13. Healthcare workers are at risk of ....
    a. Hepatitis A
    b. Hepatitis B
    c. Hepatitis D
    d. Hepatitis E

14. ....is more common in children
    a. Hepatitis A
    b. Hepatitis B
    c. Hepatitis D
    d. Hepatitis E

15. Which of the following is true about cirrhosis of the liver?

a. It is caused by a virus in the blood cells

b. Hepatitis D is a common cause

c. Blood flow through the liver is blocked

d. Signs occur at onset

16. Which of the following should be done when caring for a person with cirrhosis?

a. Measure vital signs every 2 to 4 hours

b. Apply lotion to the skin

c. Weigh the person daily

d. All of the above

17. Which of the following is a complication from liver cirrhosis?

a. Blood vessels in the stomach enlarge and burst

b. Toxics build up in the brain

c. Liver cancer may arise

d. All of the above

18. Which of the following is true about type 1diabetes?

a. It is more common in adults

b. Onset is slow

c. It is more common in whites than non-whites

d. The pancreas secretes insulin in normal quantity

19. ....develops during pregnancy

a. Type 1 diabetes

b. Type 2 diabetes

c. Gestational diabetes

d. All of the above

20. Which of the following is a sign of diabetes?

a. Blurred vision

b. Urinating often

c. Itchy skin

d.   All of the above

Section 44

Urinary and reproductive disorders

1. Urine passes from the body through the ....

a. Meatus

b. Urethra

c. Ureter

d. Bladder

2. Which of the following is true about urinary tract infection?

a. Men are at high risk

b. Prostrate gland secretions increases the risk of the infection

c. Poor nutrition increases the risk of the infection

d. All of the above

3. Cystitis is a …….. infection

a. Ureter

b. Bladder

c. Urethra

d. Kidney

4. ……is known as scant urine

a. Pyuria

b. Oliguria

c. Dysuria

d. Hematuria

5. ……..is the inflammation of the kidney pelvis

a. Cytitis

b. Pyelonephritis

c. Postrate enlargement

d. Hematuria

6. ……….is the most common cause of pyelonephritis

a. Infection

b. Urological exams

c. Poor fluid in take

d. None of the above

7. Prostrate enlargement is common after the age of ……..

a. 30

b. 40

c. 50

d. 60

8. Which of the following is included in the care plan of a person with prostrate enlargement?

a. No heavy lifting

b. No straining to have a bowel movement

c. Drinking at least 8 cups of water daily

d. All of the above

9. …….is one of the common reasons why bladder is surgically removed

a. Cancer

b. Cystitis

c. Pyelonephritis

d. Enlarged prostrate

10. Which of the following is true about urinary diversion?

a. Pouches are drained every day

b. Empty pouches every 2 days

c. Urine drains from the stoma to the pouch

d. All of the above

11. Which of the following is true about kidney stones?

a. It is more common in black women

b. Poor fluid intake is a risk factor

c. The kidney does not function properly

d. All of the above

12. Which of the following is true about kidney failure?

a. Waste products are not removed from the blood

b. Heart failure can easily occur

c. The kidneys are severely impaired

d. All of the above

13. Which of the following is true about acute kidney failure?

a. The kidneys cannot meet the body's needs

b. Every system is affected when waste products build up in the blood

c. It is sudden

d. All of the above

14. ....uses the lining of the abdominal cavity to remove the fluid from the blood

a. Peritoneal dialysis

b. Hemodialysis

c. Chemodialysis

d. Fluid restriction

15. Which of the following is true about gonorrhea?

a. There is no symptom in men

b. Burning and pain sensation occurs

c. There is intense itching

d. There is no known cure

Section 45

Mental health problems

1. Which of the following is a cause of mental health disorder?

a. Drug or substance abuse

b. Genetics

c. Chemical imbalance

d. All of the above

2. In ....state experiences and feelings cannot be recalled

a. Conscious

b. Unconscious

c. Subconscious

d. Dead

3. Which of the following is true about ego in Freud's theory of personality development?

a. It is in the unconscious level

b. Pleasure is the focus

c. Problem solving occur

d. It is concerned with right and wrong 4. Anxiety level depends on ....

a. Stressor

b. Feelings

c. Panic

d. Defense mechanism

5. ....relieves anxiety

a. Drinking

b. Exercising

c. Smoking

d. All of the above

6. ....is the highest level of anxiety

a. Panic

b. Depression

c. Insomnia

d. Pain

7. Which of the following is a symptom of anxiety?

a. Sweating

b. Loss of appetite

c. Diarrhea

d. All of the above

8. ....means intense fear

a. Panic

b. Stress

c. Phobia

d. Anxiety

9. ....is fear of night

a. Nyctophobia

b. Pyrophobia

c. Xenophobia

d. Agoraphobia

10. Post-traumatic stress disorder can occur from which of the following events?
    a. Mugging
    b. Child abuse
    c. Kidnapping
    d. All of the above

11. ....is a state of severe mental impairment
    a. Hallucination
    b. Paranoia
    c. Psychosis
    d. Delusion

12. ....is seeing, hearing or feeling something that is not real
    a. Paranoia
    b. Hallucination
    c. Delusion of grandeur
    d. Psychosis

13. Which of the following should be done when caring for a patient with schizophrenia?
    a. Speak slowly
    b. Pretend like you are experiencing the same thing
    c. Convince the person that what she is seeing is not real
    d. All of the above

14. Which of the following is true about major depression?
    a. The person has two severe extreme moods
    b. The person experiences increased energy
    c. The person is very sad
    d. There is increased sex drive

15. In .... the person shows no regard for right and wrong
    a. Major depression disorder
    b. Bipolar disorder
    c. Antisocial personality disorder
    d. Borderline personality disorder

16. Which of the following is true about borderline personality disorder?
    a. It is more common in men
    b. Child abuse is a risk factor
    c. Morals and ethics are lacking
    d. The person has no guilt

17. Which of the following is true about alcoholism?
    a. It is a chronic disease
    b. It cannot be treated
    c. It can be cured
    d. All of the above

18. ....is the overuse of a drug for a non medical or non therapy effects
    a. Drug addiction
    b. Alcoholism
    c. Drug abuse
    d. All of the above
19. Which of the following is true about bulimia nervosa?
    a. Binge eating occurs
    b. A fat body image is felt despite being thin
    c. The person avoids meals
    d. There is intense fear of weight gain
20. Which of the following is true about suicide?
    a. Firearms is the most common method for men
    b. Poison is the most common for women
    c. More men than women die from suicide
    d. All of the above

Section 46

Confusion and dementia

1. Which of the following is a cause of confusion?
    a. Disease
    b. Infection
    c. Hearing and vision loss
    d. All of the above
2. ....is the loss of cognitive function that interferes with routine personal, social and occupational activities a. Dementia
    b. Psudodementia
    c. Delirium
    d. Cognitive impairment
3. Which of the following changes occur in the nervous system from aging?
    a. Dizziness
    b. Forgetfulness
    c. Memory is shorter
    d. All of the above
4. Which of the following is true about dementia?
    a. It is a normal part of aging
    b. Most older people have dementia
    c. It is also known as delirium
    d. All of the above

5. Which of the following is a sign of dementia?
   a. Getting lost in familiar places
   b. Taste and smell decreases
   c. Reduced blood flow to the brain
   d. Sensitivity to pain increases
6. Which of the following is a sign of delirium?
   a. Delusions
   b. Forgetting simple words
   c. Wanders from home
   d. Hallucination
7. Which of the following is true about Alzheimer's disease?
   a. It is the most common mental health problem in older persons
   b. More men have AD
   c. It is a brain disease
   d. Drug abuse is a cause of AD
8. The first symptom of AD is ....
   a. Depression
   b. Swollen limb
   c. Forgetfulness
   d. Seizure
9. Which of the following is true about mild AD?
   a. Does not recognize self
   b. Loses spark for life
   c. Has seizures
   d. Falls often
10. Which of the following is true about stage 1 of AD?
    a. Family and friends notice the problems
    b. Personality changes develop
    c. The person cannot walk without help
    d. The person does not show sign of memory problem
11. With ......the signs, symptoms and behaviors of AD increase during hour of darkness
    a. Sundowning
    b. Paranoia
    c. Catastrophic reactions
    d. Hallucinations
12. Which of the following is true about paranoia?
    a. The person sees things that are not real
    b. The person has loss of cognitive function that interferes with routine personal activities
    c. It is a type of delusion
    d. It is a normal part of aging

13. Which of the following is a catastrophic reaction?
    a. Screaming
    b. Crying
    c. Being combative
    d. All of the above
14. Which of the following should be done when communication with persons with AD and dementia?
    a. Use baby voice when talking
    b. Do not interrupt the person
    c. Present the person with many questions
    d. Do not try to reason with the person
15. Which of the following is true about validation therapy?
    a. It believes that all behaviors have meaning
    b. Attempts are not made to correct the person's thought or bring back reality
    c. Caregivers need to listen and provide empathy
    d. All the above

Section 47

Developmental disability

1. A disability occurring before the age of ....is a developmental disability
    a. 10
    b. 22
    c. 30
    d. 60
2. Which of the following can cause birth defects?
    a. Rubella
    b. Smoking
    c. Using drugs
    d. All of the above
3. Which of the following is true about intellectual disability?
    a. It occurs before the age of 30
    b. The person has low intellectual function
    c. The learning rate is faster than normal
    d. All of the above
4. A person with intellectual disability has an IQ score of about .... or below
    a. 120
    b. 110
    c. 70
    d. 5o

5. Which of the following is a cause of intellectual disability after birth?
   a. Shaken baby syndrome
   b. Abnormal genes from parents
   c. Low birth weight
   d. Error when genes combine
6. Which of the following is true about Down syndrome?
   a. The fertilized egg has 49 chromosomes
   b. It is a common genetic cause of mild to moderate intellectual disability
   c. It is the most common form of inherited intellectual disabilities
   d. All of the above
7. Which of the following features occurs in children with Down syndrome? a. Flat face
   b. Small head
   c. Large tongue
   d. All of the above
8. Which of the following is true about fragile X syndrome?
   a. It is inherited
   b. Boys often have more milder symptoms
   c. A person with fragile X syndrome cannot control muscle contractions
   d. The cause is unknown
9. Which of the following symptoms relates to fragile X syndrome?
   a. Fear and anxiety in new situations
   b. Long ears
   c. Stuttering is common among boys
   d. All of the above
10. ……..is a group of disorders involving muscle weakness or poor muscle control
    a. Fragile X syndrome
    b. Autism
    c. Cerebral palsy
    d. Spina bifida
11. Which of the following is true about a person with athetoid?
    a. The person cannot control movements
    b. The arm and leg on one side are paralyzed
    c. Muscles are stiff
    d. Joints are loosed and flexible
12. Which of the following is true about hemiplegia?
    a. The body parts on both sides are paralyzed
    b. The arm and leg on one side are paralyzed
    c. Both arms and both legs are paralyzed
    d. The trunk and the neck muscles are paralyzed 13. Which of the following is true about autism?

a. It begins in late childhood
b. It is inherited
c. It is a brain disorder
d. It involves poor muscle control

14. Which of the following is an early sign of autism?
a. Poor eye contact
b. No single word by 16 months
c. No response to his or her name
d. All of the above

15. Which of the following is true about spina bifida?
a. It is a defect in the brain
b. Cerebrospinal fluid collects in the brain
c. Bowel and bladder problems are common
d. All of the above

Section 48

Sexuality

1. The female sex glands are called the ………
a. Ovaries
b. Fallopian tube
c. Estrogen
d. Vagina

2. The…….is the male sex organ
a. Scrotum
b. Testes
c. Sperm
d. Testosterone

3. Sexuality is shown in……….
a. Color
b. Toys
c. Names
d. All of the above

4. Which of the following is true about sexuality?
a. It starts to develop in the teenage years
b. Teens are more aware of sex and the body
c. It does not involve a person's personality
d. All of the above

5. A ……….is a person who is attracted to members of the other sex

a. Heterosexual
b. Homosexual
c. Bisexual
d. Transvestites

6. ....are persons who dress and behave like the other sex for emotional and sexual relief
   a. Transsexuals
   b. Transvestites
   c. Trans-dressers
   d. Transgender

7. Which of the following is true about transsexuals?
   a. They usually dress as women in private
   b. They believe they are members of the opposite sex
   c. They are attracted to both sexes
   d. They take part in cross dressing

8. Which of the following illnesses affects sexual function?
   a. Heart disease
   b. Stroke
   c. Diabetes
   d. All of the above

9. All of the following should be done to promote sexuality EXCEPT?
   a. Select appropriate clothing for the person
   b. Allow privacy for masturbation
   c. Protect do not judge relationships
   d. Allow the person practice grooming routines

10. Which of the following is a cause of sexually aggressive behavior?
    a. Fever
    b. Nervous system disorders
    c. Poor vision
d.   All of the above

Section 49

Caring for mothers and newborns

1. Babies ....to communicate
   a. Cry

b. Moan

c. Groan

d. Move

2. Babies feel secure when ....

    a. Sleeping

    b. Warm and held

    c. Eating

    d. Crying

3. Which of the following safety guidelines should be followed when caring for babies?

    a. The only jewelry to be worn is a ring

    b. Shake powders gently over the baby

    c. Restrain the baby in the car seats

    d. Tie a pacifier loosely around the baby's neck 4. When holding a baby, ...

    a. Lift the new born by the arms

    b. Use both hands to lift the new born

    c. Neck support should be given for at least 2 weeks after birth

    d. All of the above

5. Which of the following safety measure should be followed in crib safety?

    a. Lay infant on soft bedding products

    b. Place crib away from heat sources

    c. Place soft pillows in the crib

    d. Place soft toys in the crib

6. Which of the following is a sign of illness in babies?

    a. The baby looks sick

    b. The baby has rash

    c. The baby is less active

    d. All of the above

7. Which of the following should be done when helping with breast-feeding?

    a. Help lay the baby on the stomach

    b. Soap should be used to clean the breast and nipples

    c. Encourage the mother to wear nursing bra

    d. All of the above

8. Which of the following should be part of a nursing mother's nutrition?

    a. 3 servings a day from milk

    b. Caffeine

    c. Alcohol

    d. Spices

9. Which of the following is true about ready to feed formulas?

    a. Contents should be use after 48 hours of opening

    b. Container directions explain how much liquid to use

c. It is poured from can into baby bottle

d. All of the above

10. Which of the following is true about a baby's bowel movement?

    a. Bottle fed babies have yellow and seedy looking stools

    b. Bottle fed babies have more stools than breast fed babies

    c. Bottle fed babies have firmer stools

d.   Breast fed babies have stools 1 or 2 times a day

Section 50

Assisted living

1. Assisted living residence usually offers all of the following EXCEPT

    a. 1 meal a day

    b. Transportation

    c. Exercise and wellness program

    d. 24 hour security

2. Which of the following is a requirement and feature of assisted living units? a. A television

    b. Spa and gym facilities

    c. A telephone jack

    d. Barbeque stand

3. Which of the following is an environment requirement of assisted living unit?

    a. The ALR be free of rodents and insects

    b. The ALR is clean, safe, and orderly

    c. The hot and cold water supply meets hygiene needs

    d. All of the above

4. ALR have which of the following rights?

    a. To terminate living at an ARL after 2 days written notice if the ARL failed to comply with the service plan or residency agreement

    b. To decide how the ALR will be managed

    c. To make choices about how to receive care

    d. To determine how the ALR will be designed

5. The assisted living residents have right to be free from ………

    a. Involuntary seclusion

    b. Chemical restraints

    c. Discrimination

    d. All of the above

6. A ………is a written plan listing services needed, how much help is needed and who provides the service a. Nursing plan

    b. Service plan

    c. Tenancy agreement

d. Daily plan

7. Which of the following is a staff requirement
    a. Must not have a criminal record
    b. Must be older than 21
    c. Must be a registered nurse
    d. All of the above

8. Which of the following should be practiced to ensure food safety?
    a. Use left over food within 1 week
    b. Towel dry after washing cooking items
    c. Use liquid detergent and hot water for washing dishes
    d. Empty garbage every 3 days

9. Which of the following house keeping measures should be taken to prevent infection?
    a. Dust furniture at least weekly as needed
    b. Sweep daily or as needed
    c. Clean the tub or shower after use
    d. All of the above

10. When helping with drug administration, ensure that the right ……. Is used
    a. Drug
    b. Dosage
    c. Route
    d. All of the above

Section 51

Basic emergency care

1. …….is the emergency care given to an ill or injured person before medical help arrives a. First aid
    b. Mouth resuscitation
    c. Giving abdominal thrust
    d. None of the above

2. The goal of first aid is to ……
    a. Prevent death
    b. Cure sickness
    c. Treat illness
    d. All of the above

3. Which of the following rules should be followed in case of emergency?
    a. Move the person away from onlookers
    b. Remove the person's clothes
    c. Check for life threatening problems

d. Give the person some food

4. ....is when the heart stops suddenly and without warning
    a. Respiratory arrest
    b. Sudden cardiac arrest
    c. Fainting
    d. Stroke

5. Which of the following is a major sign of cardiac arrest?
    a. No response
    b. No breathing
    c. No pulse
    d. All of the above

6. ....is a cause of cardiac arrest
    a. Electric shock
    b. High fever
    c. Paralysis
    d. Lupus

7. ....is when breathing stops but heart actions continues for several minutes
    a. Dyspnea
    b. Apnea
    c. Respiratory arrest
    d. Cardiac arrest

8. Rescue breathing is given when ....
    a. There is no pulse and no breathing
    b. There is a pulse but no breathing
    c. There no pulse or grasping
    d. The hearts stops suddenly and there is no pulse

9. To find the carotid pulse, place 2 or 3 finger tips on the ....
    a. Chest
    b. Inner wrist
    c. Trachea
    d. Elbow

10. Check for a pulse for at least ....
    a. 5 seconds
    b. 12 seconds
    c. 15 seconds
    d. 20 seconds

11. Which of the following should be used for chest compressions?
    a. The knuckles
    b. The fist
    c. The heel of the hands
    d. The palm

12. The AHA recommends which of the following?

a. Give compressions at a rate of 100 per minute

b. Push hard and push fast

c. Push deeply into the chest

d. All of the above

13. Which of the following should be done when giving mouth-to-mouth breathing?

   a. Use your thumb to raise the lower jaw

   b. Take a deep breath

   c. Blow air into the person's mouth

   d. Keep the nostrils open

14. Mouth to nose is done when ....

   a. You cannot open the mouth

   b. Your mouth is too small to make a tight seal for mouth-to-mouth breathing

   c. The mouth or jaw is severely injured

   d. All of the above

15. When giving mouth to stoma breathing,.........

   a. Keep the mouth opened

   b. Seal your mouth around the stoma

   c. Tilt the person's head back

   d. All of the above

16. Which of the following is true about defibrillation?

   a. It is used to deliver shock to the heart

   b. For adults manual defibrillation is the best

   c. The shock dosage for children 4 years and older is the same as adult dosage

   d. All of the above

17. Which of the following is a CPR rule for infants

   a. Use the 2 thumbs encircling hands method for chest compressions when there are 2 rescuers

   b. Give compressions at a rate of at least 100 per minute

   c. Use the brachial artery to check for a pulse

   d. All of the above

18. To control external bleeding, ...

   a. Remove the pierced object

   b. Apply pressure for one minute directly over the bleeding site then remove hand

   c. Bind the wound when bleeding stops

   d. Give fluids and food immediately

19. ....is the sudden loss of consciousness from an inadequate blood supply to the brain

   a. Shock

b. Fainting

c. Stroke

d. Death

20. Which of the following is a sign of shock?

    a. Weak pulse

    b. Rapid respirations

    c. Low blood pressure

    d. All of the above

Section 52

End of life care

1. An illness or injury from which the person will not likely recover is a ……….

    a. Acute illness

    b. Chronic illness

    c. Terminal illness

    d. Tragic illness

2. Which of the following is true about hospice care?

    a. The goal is to improve quality of life

    b. Pain relief is stressed

    c. Often the person has less than 6 months to live

    d. All of the above

3. The first stage of death is …….

    a. Denial

    b. Depression

    c. Anger

    d. Bargaining

4. Which of the following occurs in stage 2 of death?

    a. The person refuses to believe he or she is dying

    b. The person is calm and at peace

    c. The person is angry and envious

    d. The person begins to mourn

5. Which of the following is the last stage of death

    a. Depression

    b. Acceptance

    c. Bargaining

    d. Anger

6. Which of the following is an important part of end-of-life care?

    a. Listening to the person

b. Touching to show care

c. Giving spiritual needs

d. All of the above

7. Which of the following helps to prevent breathing problems?

a. Placing the person in a prone position

b. Carrying out suctioning by the nurse

c. Ensuring that the room is cold

d. All of the above

8. ....is a document stating a person's wishes about health care when that person cannot make his or her own decisions a. An advance directive

b. Living wills

c. Wills

d. Do not resuscitate orders

9. Which of the following is a sign of death?

a. Drowsiness

b. Shortness of breath

c. Confusion

d. All of the above

10. Rigor mortis develops within ......after death

a. 20 minutes

b. 35 minutes

c. 40 minutes

d. 2 hours

ANSWERS

Section 1

Introduction to care agencies

1. D
2. C
3. A
4. B
5. A
6. A
7. C
8. B
9. D
10. B
11. C
12. D
13. B
14. C
15. A
16. A
17. D
18. C
19. B
20. B
21. A
22. C
23. B
24. C
25. B
26. A
27. D
28. D
29. C
30. A
31. C
32. B
33. B
34. D
35. D
36. B
37. C

38. D
39. C
40. D

Section 2

The person's rights

1. D
2. A
3. D
4. D
5. B
6. A
7. C
8. D
9. D
10. A
11. C
12. A
13. C
14. C

15. B

Section 3

The nursing assistant

1. C
2. D
3. D
4. A
5. C
6. A
7. B
8. D
9. C
10. A
11. B
12. D

13. A

14. B 15. C

Section 4

Ethics and laws

1. B
2. D
3. A
4. C
5. A
6. D
7. D
8. A
9. B
10. C
11. D
12. B
13. C
14. A
15. B
16. C
17. D
18. D
19. B
20. A

Section 5

Work ethics

1. D
2. A
3. B
4. D
5. C
6. D
7. B
8. A
9. A
10. C

11. A
12. A
13. B
14. C
15. D

Section 6

Communicating with the health team

1. B
2. A
3. B
4. C
5. D
6. C
7. B
8. A
9. B
10. C
11. C
12. A
13. A
14. D
15. D

Section 7

Assisting with the nursing process

1. A
2. C
3. C
4. D
5. A
6. A
7. C
8. A
9. D

10. D

Section 8

Understanding the person

1. A
2. D
3. B
4. C
5. D
   6.   B

7. C
8. A
9. B
10. A
11. C
12. A
13. C
14. A
15. D
16. A
17. C
18. C
19. A
20. B

Section 9

Body structure and function

1. A
2. B
3. A
4. C
5. C
6. A
7. B
8. B
9. A
10. C
11. D
12. B
13. C
14. A
15. B
16. C
17. D
18. B
19. D
20. D
21. B

22. A
23. C
24. A
25. B
26. D
27. C
28. A
29. B
30. C
31. C
32. B
33. A
34. C
35. A
36. D
37. D
38. C
39. A
40. C
41. B
42. D
43. B
44. A
45. B
46. C
47. A
48. B
49. C
50. B

Section 10

Growth and development

1. D
2. C
3. A
4. D
5. A
6. B

7. D
8. B
9. C
10. B
11. D
12. D
13. A
14. C
15. C
16. D
17. D
18. A
19. B
20. C
21. D
22. A
23. B
24. D
25. D

Section 11

Care of the older person

1. D
2. A
3. B
4. D
5. B
6. C
7. C
8. C
9. A
10. D
11. B
12. D

13. A
14. C
15. D

Section 12

Safety

1. A
2. D
3. C
4. B
5. D
    6.   C
    7.   D
    8.   A
    9.   A
    10.   **B**

    11. C
    12. D
    13. D
    14. A
    15. B
    16. A
    17. C
    18. C
    19. A
    20. D

Section 13

Preventing falls

1. D
2. B
3. C
4. D
5. A
6. A
7. B

8. C
9. C
10. A

Section 14

Restraint alternatives and safe restraint use

1. B
2. D
3. C
4. A
5. B
6. D
7. A
8. C
9. C
10. C
11. A
12. B
13. D
14. D
15. C
16. B
17. A
18. A
19. D

20. B

Section 15

Preventing infection

1. D
2. D
3. A
4. B
5. C

6. B
7. A
8. A
9. B
10. C
11. D
12. B
13. A
14. B
15. D
16. B
17. C
18. D
19. B
20. A
21. C
22. C
23. A
24. D
25. D
26. A
27. B
28. C
29. A
30. D

Section 16

Body mechanism

1. D
2. A
3. C
4. A
5. B
6. C
7. D
8. D
9. A
10. C

Section 17

Safely moving and transferring the person

1. D
2. A
3. C
4. B
5. B
6. A
7. C
8. A
9. B
10. C
11. B
12. C
13. A
14. B
15. A
16. C
17. B
18. D
19. C
20. A

Section 18

The person's unit

1. A
2. C
3. D
4. A
5. D
6. B
7. C
8. D
9. B
10. A
11. C

12. A
13. C
14. A
15. D
16. D
17. C
18. A
19. A

20. B

Section 19

Bedmaking

1. A
2. B
3. C
4. C
5. C
6. A
7. C
8. B
9. B
10. D
11. D
12. B
13. D
14. A

15. D

Section 20

Personal hygiene

1. A
2. D
3. B
4. D
5. D

6. B
7. C
8. C
9. D
10. A
11. D
12. C
13. A
14. B
15. D
16. C
17. B
18. C
19. C
20. D
21. A
22. C
23. D
24. A

25. D

Section 21

Grooming

1. A
2. D
3. B
4. C
5. A
6. D
7. A
8. B
9. A
10. A
11. C
12. D
13. C

14. C
15. A
16. B
17. D
18. C
19. B

20. C

Section 22

Urinary elimination

1. B
2. C
3. B
4. D
5. A
6. A
7. C
8. D
9. D
10. B
11. A
12. C
13. D
14. B
15. A
16. D
17. A
18. B
19. C
20. D
21. A
22. C
23. B
24. A

25. D

Section
23

Bowel elimination

1. D
2. C
3. C
4. B
5. B
6. C
7. D
8. A
9. D
10. A
11. D
12. C
13. D
14. A
15. B
16. A
17. C
18. D
19. A

20. 20. C

Section 24

Nutrition and fluids

1. D
2. A
3. C
4. B
5. A
6. C
7. C
8. B
9. D
10. B
11. A

12. D
13. C
14. C
15. D
16. B
17. C
18. A
19. A
20. B
21. D
22. B
23. C
24. B
25. A
26. D
27. B
28. D
29. B
30. D

Section 25

Nutritional support and IV therapy

1. D
2. B
3. A
4. A
5. A
6. C
7. C
8. D
9. B
10. C
11. D
12. B
13. A
14. B
15. C
16. D
17. A
18. B

19. C

20. D

Section 26

Measuring vital signs

1. D
2. D
3. C
4. A
5. C
6. C
7. B
8. D
9. A
10. A
11. C
12. B
13. A
14. B
15. C
16. D
17. C
18. B
19. C

20. D

Section 27

Exercise and activity

1. D
2. A
3. D
4. A
5. C

6. B
7. B
8. A
9. A
10. C
11. A
12. B
13. C
14. D
15. C

Section 28

Comfort, Rest and sleep

1. B
2. A
3. C
4. C
5. A
6. D
7. C
8. D
9. C
10. A
11. D
12. B
13. B
14. C
15. C

Section 29

Admission, Transfers and Discharges

1. B
2. B
3. B

4. D
5. D
6. B
7. A
8. A
9. D
10. B

Section 30

Assisting with physical examination

1. D
2. B
3. C
4. C
5. A
6. B
7. D
8. A
9. B
10. C
11. A
12. C
13. D
14. D
15. C

Section 31

Collecting and testing specimens

1. D
2. C
3. D
4. A
5. B
6. A
7. B
8. C

9. D
10. A
11. B
12. D
13. C
14. A
15. A
16. C
17. C
18. B
19. B
20. D

Section 32

The person having surgery

1. D
2. C
3. C
4. A
5. D
6. A
7. B
8. A
9. C
10. C
11. B
12. B
13. D
14. A
15. A
16. B
17. C
18. A
19. B
20. C
21. A
22. D

23. A
24. B
25. C
26. D
27. C
28. B
29. A
30. D

Section 33

Wound care

1. B
2. C
3. B
4. A
5. D
6. A
7. C
8. A
9. C
10. D
11. D
12. B
13. C
14. B
15. A
16. D
17. C
18. A
19. B
20. C
21. A
22. A
23. A
24. C
25. B
26. D
27. D
28. A

29. D 30. C

Section 34

Pressure ulcers

1. A
2. B
3. B
4. D
5. C
6. A
7. C
8. A
9. B
10. C
11. B
12. A
13. C
14. A
15. B

Section 35

Heat and cold applications

1. D
2. C
3. A
4. D
5. A
6. B
7. C
8. C
9. D
10. B

Section 36

Oxygen needs

1. D
2. A
3. B
4. D
5. A
6. D
7. A
8. C
9. B
10. A
11. C
12. B
13. D
14. A
15. B
16. D
17. C
18. D
19. D
20. D
21. A
22. B
23. D
24. C
25. A

Sections 37

Respiratory support and therapies

1. A
2. B
3. B
4. D
5. C
6. C

7. A
8. D
9. B
10. C
11. D
12. A
13. A
14. B
15. D

Section 38

Rehabilitation and restorative nursing care

1. B
2. D
3. C
4. A
5. A
6. C
7. B
8. D
9. D
10. A

Section 39

Hearing, speech and vision problems

1. D
2. A
3. B
4. C
5. B
6. B
7. A
8. D
9. A
10. C
11. B

12. C
13. B
14. A
15. A
16. D
17. C
18. D
19. A
20. D
21. B
22. B
23. D
24. C
25. A
26. C
27. B
28. D
29. A
30. A
31. B
32. D
33. C
34. D
35. C
36. D
37. A
38. B
39. B
40. C

Section 40

Cancer, immune system, skin disorder

1. B
2. A
3. D
4. C
5. C
6. A
7. B
8. D

9. D
10. D
11. A
12. C
13. A
14. B
15. C
16. A
17. B
18. C
19. B
20. A
21. D
22. D
23. B
24. D
25. C

Section 41

Nervous system and musculo skeletal disorders

1. A
2. B
3. D
4. C
5. D
6. B
7. A
8. C
9. D
10. B
11. C
12. A
13. D
14. B
15. A
16. C
17. B

18. D
19. D
20. A

Section 42

Cardiovascular, respiratory and lymphatic disorder

1. D
2. D
3. C
4. B
5. A
6. D
7. A
8. C
9. B
10. C
11. A
12. D
13. D
14. A
15. B
16. A
17. C
18. A
19. B
20. D

Section 43

Digestive and endocrine disorders

1. A
2. D
3. D
4. C
5. B
6. D

7. A
8. B
9. A
10. B
11. D
12. A
13. B
14. A
15. C
16. D
17. D
18. C
19. C
20. D

Section 44

Urinary and reproductive disorders

1. A
2. C
3. B
4. B
5. B
6. A
7. D
8. D
9. A
10. C
11. B
12. D
13. C
14. A
15. B

Section 45

Mental health problems

1. D
2. B
3. C
4. A
5. D
6. A
7. D
8. C
9. A
10. D
11. C
12. B
13. A
14. C
15. C
16. B
17. A
18. C
19. A
20. D

Section 46

Confusion and dementia

1. D
2. A
3. D
4. B
5. A
6. B
7. C
8. C
9. B
10. D
11. A
12. C

13. D
14. B
15. D

Section 47

Developmental disability

1. B
2. D
3. B
4. C
5. A
6. B
7. D
8. A
9. D
10. C
11. A
12. B
13. C
14. D
15. C

Section 48

Sexuality

1. A
2. B
3. C
4. B
5. B
6. D
7. C
8. A
9. C
10. C

11. B
12. D
13. A
14. D

Section 49

Caring for mothers and newborns

1. A
2. B
3. C
4. B
5. B
6. D
7. C
8. A
9. C
10. C

Section 50

Assisted living

1. A
2. C
3. D
4. C
5. D
6. B
7. A
8. C
9. D
10. D

Section 51

Basic emergency care

1. A
2. A
3. C
4. B
5. D
6. A
7. C
8. B
9. C
10. A
11. C
12. D
13. C
14. D
15. B
16. A
17. D
18. C
19. B

20. D

Section 52

End of life care

1. C
2. D
3. A
4. C
5. B
6. D

7. B
8. A
9. D
10. D

www.ingramcontent.com/pod-product-compliance
Lightning Source LLC
Chambersburg PA
CBHW081724220526
45468CB00008B/1963